Working Happy!

*How to Survive Burnout and
Find Your Work/Life Synergy
in the Healthcare Industry*

Roger Kapoor, MD, MBA

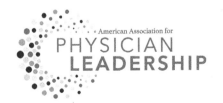

American Association for
PHYSICIAN
LEADERSHIP

Published by **American Association for Physician Leadership, Inc.**
PO Box 96503 | BMB 97493 | Washington, DC 20090-6503

Website: www.physicianleaders.org

AAPL books are available at special quantity discounts to use as premiums and sales promotions, or for use in corporate training programs. For more information, please write to Special Sales at journal@physicianleaders.org

This publication is designed to provide general information and is sold with the understanding that neither the author nor the publisher is engaged in rendering legal, accounting, ethical, or clinical advice. If legal or other expert advice is required, the services of a competent professional person should be sought.

13   8 7 6 5 4 3 2 1

Copyedited, typeset, indexed, and printed in the United States of America

PUBLISHER
Nancy Collins

PRODUCTION MANAGER
Jennifer Weiss

DESIGN & LAYOUT
Carter Publishing Studio

COPYEDITOR
Patricia George

This book is dedicated to my loving wife, supportive family, colleagues, and to all the aspiring doctors and leaders who strive to make a difference.

Table of Contents

Preface xi

Introduction xiii

CHAPTER 1

Unhappy Workers and Employee Burnout 1

  The Creeping Malaise | 4

  A Global Burnout Epidemic | 5

CHAPTER 2

The Two Sources of Burnout 11

  Your Stressful Workplace | 12

    Having Little or No Control Over Your Work | 14

    Lack of Recognition | 15

    Lofty Goal Setting / Performance Expectations | 15

    Monotonous or Unchallenging Work | 16

    Chaotic Environment | 17

    Toxic Culture | 18

  Your Own Lifestyle | 21

    All Work and No Play | 21

    Lack of Close, Supportive Relationships | 22

    Biting Off More Than You Can Chew | 23

    Not Enough Sleep | 23

    Perfectionistic Tendencies | 24

    Need to Be in Control | 26

    Unreasonable Rigidity | 29

    Survivor's Guilt | 30

CHAPTER 3

Finding Work/Life Synergy 33

  Is It Your Job or Your Career? | 35

    Look Beyond Today's Paycheck | 36

Ask Yourself What You Would Do if Every Job
  Paid the Same | 39

Identify the Source of Your Pain | 40

CHAPTER 4

Path #1: Find Happiness in Your Present Job **45**

Make Change Within Your Company | 45

Working Happy Through Adversity | 49

Make Change Within Yourself | 51

Become an "Organization Person" | 51

CHAPTER 5

Path #2: Change Jobs **57**

Finding a Company You Like | 61

  Google Them! | 62

  Glassdoor | 62

  Indeed | 63

CHAPTER 6

Path #3: Change Your Career **65**

The Four Reasons People Change Careers | 67

  1. They're Burned Out | 67

  2. They've Gone as Far as Their Current Career Can Take
    Them | 68

  3. They "Age Out" of a Successful Career | 69

  4. They Need New Challenges | 70

Add a Side Venture or Productive Hobby | 71

Know Your Desired Future State | 73

Look at the Big Picture | 74

Money and Training | 76

An Unsatisfied Affinity: The Career Journey of Vera
Wang | 78

CHAPTER 7

Emotional Resilience **85**

Optimism | 88

Emotional Intelligence | 90

   1. Self-Awareness | 90

   2. Self-Management | 93

   3. Social Awareness | 94

   4. Relationship Management | 94

Internal Locus of Control | 95

Hedonic and Eudaimonic Well-Being | 97

Perseverance | 98

Sense of Humor | 99

Willingness to Face Your Fears | 101

Rest and Recover | 102

Take a Time Out | 104

Make a Personal Checklist | 105

CHAPTER 8

Self-Help Strategies: Make Small Changes **109**

Free Yourself from Distractions | 110

Exercise Your Right to Disconnect | 113

Be Kind to Yourself | 114

No More Workcations, Wolidays, Bleisure Travel... | 115

Manage Expectations | 118

Keep It Real | 119

The Power of Gratitude | 120

Better Inputs = Better Outputs | 122

The Company You Keep | 123

The Power of Words | 125

CHAPTER 9

Your Purpose in Work and Life **129**

Your Purpose | 132

A Word About Money as a Motivator | 135

Overcome Your Fear of the Future | 139

Ikigai — Your "Life-Value" | 142

CHAPTER 10

Keep Working Happy! 145

Your Diet, Weight, and Health | 145

Meditation | 152

Exercise | 154

Lifelong Learning | 156

Volunteer in Service to Others | 158

Thank You! 163

References 165

Acknowledgments

Writing a book is not a solitary endeavor and I am deeply grateful to everyone who has played a part in bringing this work to fruition.

To Nancy Collins, a truly remarkable and dedicated individual, and the entire publishing team, thank you for your expertise, dedication, and tireless efforts. Your commitment to excellence is inspiring.

About the Author

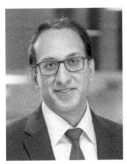

Roger Kapoor, MD, is the senior vice president of Beloit Health System in Beloit, Wisconsin, a community-based nonprofit hospital with approximately 23 service locations.

A Harvard-trained dermatologist, he holds an MBA from Oxford University in England and has authored numerous peer-reviewed scientific articles published in professional journals, including The *New England Journal of Medicine*. He was the recipient of the Wisconsin Medical Society's Kenneth M. Viste Young Physician Leader of the Year Award and named by *Modern Healthcare* as one of the top 25 Emerging Leaders in Healthcare.

Kapoor has been credited for re-engineering the delivery of healthcare to his community, resulting in a dramatic rise in patient satisfaction at his institution from a stagnant 16th percentile to an astonishing 88th percentile in less than a year.

He concurrently ushered in transformative results in quality, leading teams to achieve three consecutive "A" ratings from the national watchdog group Leapfrog, a 4-star rating from the Center for Medicare and Medicaid Services Quality Star program, and numerous quality-of-care pathway accolades.

As a practicing board-certified dermatologist, he has built a successful medical and cosmetic dermatology practice using advanced techniques to help patients live happier, healthier lives.

He and his wife have two children and live in Beloit, Wisconsin.

PREFACE

I HAD REACHED MY BREAKING POINT.

Two years out of residency, feeling drained and disillusioned, I found myself drowning under the incessant demands of my medical career. The once bright flame of passion for healing had dimmed, suffocated by tedious administrative tasks, long hours, the continuous adoption of new electronic medical record upgrades, a focus by management on my patient satisfaction score, and a sense of disconnection from the very purpose that had drawn me into medicine.

It was on one of those miserable days in my office that I opened the door to the exam room to see a new patient: a 17-year-old girl with her mother.

"What brought you in today?" I asked the mother.

"Routine skin exam," she replied. "Lily is a lifeguard, and my father had melanoma."

"Better to be safe than sorry," I said.

At the end of my evaluation, I sat down with Lily and her mother and, as usual, began to review my findings. I had identified a small mole with irregular borders that I felt warranted further evaluation. After a discussion, we agreed to a skin biopsy.

A few days later, her pathology report came back: invasive malignant melanoma. As gently as I could, I told Lily and her mother the diagnosis. This was an emotional moment, but they both put on a brave face and agreed to aggressively fight the disease.

Lily began rounds of radiation and chemotherapy treatments. We stayed in close contact, and when I would call to check in on how she was doing, she always remained positive, even when I was starting to become less optimistic about her diagnosis.

Sadly, after a period in intensive care, Lily passed away.

I was humbled to be asked to speak at Lily's funeral. Her mother revealed to me that in her daughter's final days, Lily had spoken about how I had become a pillar of emotional support during her challenging journey. As time passed, I began to realize the profound impact that Lily had on me. She had reignited my appreciation for the sacred space created when genuine human connection is made — a space where compassion, empathy, and understanding can and will flourish.

Lily reminded me of the profound impact a physician can have not just on a patient's disease but on their life, and the immense privilege it is to be entrusted with their care.

Buoyed by this renewed sense of purpose, I sought out connections with my patients, engaged in open conversations, truly listened to their concerns, and tailored my care to their unique needs. And as I was doing these things, something changed within me. Gradually, the stress that I had been feeling began to melt away. I began to feel truly happy, that my work meant something and was valuable.

The change was not instantaneous; I didn't suddenly wake up one day willing to embrace the same old stress I had been experiencing. The change influenced how I approached my work and helped me prioritize and become more efficient. It changed not only how I *felt* about my job but how I *did* my job. With the feeling in my heart that I truly made a difference to my patients, I got better at pursuing the goal of healing without getting tangled up in things that didn't matter.

I wrote this book to share my journey and the insights that I've gained along the way, bolstered by the wisdom of many caring colleagues and friends. Indeed, while this book is written from the perspective of the healthcare industry, its principles can be applied to anyone who works for a living and who has, at some point in their lives, asked themselves, "Why am I killing myself for this job?"

The answer — as I found out — might be that you're in the wrong job, but it could also be that you're not seeing your current job in the best way. If you could learn to see both yourself and your job in the best possible light, I think you'd have a very good chance to be Working Happy!

INTRODUCTION

How do you feel about your work and your life?

I'm not asking how much you get paid or if you're successful. You could be at any stage of your healthcare career: beginning, middle, or nearing retirement. The question is, when you leave your home to go to your workplace every day, do you go with a happy heart or with drudgery and maybe even some loathing? When you come home after a full day or shift at work, do you feel pleased with what you've accomplished or grateful to be free from that horrible place of endless toil?

Many people would balk at that question. They would reply, "Who really is happy at work? It's just a means to an end that drains you of time and energy and something all grown-ups must endure. That's why you have weekends to look forward to!"

I have good news: It doesn't have to be that way. Do you ever wonder about that "odd" individual who actually seems to be *happy* at work and home? You likely tell yourself it's a façade, but deep down, you know that it's true and wonder how he or she is managing it. The reality is that you *deserve* to have a happy life at work and at home. Plenty of other people just like you enjoy their work and their home life. They don't suffer from workplace burnout, and you don't have to either.

The title of this book is *Working Happy! How to Survive Burnout and Find Your Work/Life Synergy in the Healthcare Industry*. My hope is that this book can help you change how you feel about your work and your life.

The title encompasses three ideas. They're all interconnected and express three different aspects of the same goal for your life.

The first is the idea of "working happy." I've combined these words deliberately. In some capacity, we all perform a task that may seem trivial at the time, but at its core, we may not always recognize that the ultimate purpose of work is *the pursuit of happiness*. Whether you work in a home, a hospital, a remote clinic, or a gleaming office tower, you're almost certainly engaged in a productive activity that not only pays the bills but also should give you a sense of fulfillment along the path of your pursuit of happiness. Whether you decided to go to school, pursue a particular job, or have a family, it was because you felt that these decisions would make you happy. Undeniably, the work done by the human species, collectively and over time, has resulted in an incredible amount of comfort and convenience that even kings and queens from the past might not even imagine. But with all of that convenience, are we any happier?

When we say "happy," we mean a condition that's sustainable and not transient. Sadly, too many people, perhaps even you, find their work to be boring, aggravating, stressful, emotionally painful — any number of descriptors that are not "happy." We have all experienced moments of happiness, but the problem is that for a variety of reasons, we are not able to sustain it. Among other messages I hope to deliver in this book is the idea that not only *can* work be happy, but it *should* be happy, and you can *make it* happy — permanently! You deserve to go to work every day with a glad heart and return home feeling just as good as when you left.

The second idea in the title is "burnout." This happens when unhappy feelings persist over time. It's one thing to have a bad day at work — we all do occasionally — but if you have bad days that stretch into weeks and then months, you have a problem. You're going to dread going to work every day, and when you're there, you'll be watching the clock for when you can go home. This is not a good situation for anybody, including your employer and your customers. It can lead to personal stagnation and, in severe cases, even self-medication with alcohol or drugs.

As we'll see in the pages ahead, workplace burnout is a serious problem throughout the industrialized world, including the healthcare industry, and you need to know how to avoid it.

The third idea in the title is "work/life synergy." This may sound similar to the familiar expression "work/life balance," but as the book reveals, there's a key difference. The word "balance" implies two different things that should be of equal weight, as if they were on a set of scales. You have your work on one side of the scale and your life outside of work on the other side, and you are struggling to balance them. Balanced, but not blended. This image conjures the vision of the 1960s doctor who lives in suburbia, commutes to work every morning, puts in his eight hours, and drives home. When he gets home, he takes off his suit and tie and relaxes with a martini. On weekends he dons a polo shirt and plays golf. Work and life — two separate worlds.

On the other hand, the word "synergy" is much more dynamic. It means an interaction or cooperation of two or more entities to produce a combined effect greater than the sum of them in isolation. In other words, if you have work/life synergy, your life does not merely *tolerate* your work, and vice-versa. It's not a question of peaceful co-existence between the two, whereby they neither damage nor benefit each other. It's something much better. Magically now, it's like 2 + 2 = 5.

Think about this for a moment. You — and every human being — get just one life. You get your 80 or 90 years on earth, and you want to make the most of it. How dreary would life be if the highest level you could attain was an amicable work/life balance? Or a polite cease-fire between your work and your life? Don't you think you — and everyone — should aspire to more? Aspire to a life where both things work symbiotically to make you truly happy and fulfilled for every moment of your life?

The goal of this book is to help you bring these two arenas — your work and your life — together to make a stronger and more uplifting result, one in which the lines between your work and life are pleasantly blurred and you don't feel any tension between the two.

We'll begin by revealing just how serious a problem workplace burnout is. This will reassure you that if you feel burned out or as if your work and life were separated by a wide chasm, you are not alone, and you can find the solution.

You can't hope to defeat burnout unless you know how it's created, so we reveal the two sources of burnout. The first (no surprise here) is your workplace, but the second (surprise!) may very well be your own lifestyle and attitudes. Remember, workplace dissatisfaction — the root of burnout — comes from a misalignment of your *propensities* and *reality*. The bigger the gap between them, the more likely there is to be burnout. By committing just a few basic mistakes, such as depriving yourself of sleep or driving yourself too hard, you can contribute to your own workplace burnout.

We'll look at the work you do and ask you, "If you could do your job with no regard for the money, would you still do it?" So many famous achievers who have enjoyed a positive work/life synergy have said that they think their work is fun and would do it even if they weren't getting paid. Could you say that?

The criteria for your happiness must not be related to whether the work seems hard. In fact, one of the interesting things about people who love their work and have a good work/life synergy is that they often work harder and longer at their jobs than people who are disengaged. When you love what you do, you'll find that working long hours comes naturally, without any particular extra effort.

I'll ask you if you've truly done all you can do to find happiness in your present job. Is there anything you could change about yourself or your role to find greater happiness?

You may have no choice but to look for another job with a different organization. This is a case whereby you enjoy your career path but are a poor fit at your particular company. That can be okay; there's no law that says you must be happy working for a company that you might have chosen randomly because you needed a job or because they hired you arbitrarily to fill a position.

Despite your efforts to find happiness in your present industry, your dissatisfaction may run deep, and you may be looking to change not just your job but also your career path. In this case, you may have what I call an unsatisfied affinity: a strong interest in a field or vocation that you're not working in. In one of the dozens of true-life case studies in the book, we'll look at the fascinating life of Vera Wang, who went from Olympic figure skating hopeful to fashion magazine editor to the founder of her hugely successful bridal and couture design house.

Your job and career are only one side of the work/life synergy equation. This book provides you with a robust toolkit of techniques and approaches that can help you lower your stress level and recognize a new dimension of work/life synergy you might not have known could exist. We'll talk about how to strengthen your emotional resilience, boost your optimism, face your fears, and take a "time out" when you need to recharge.

Most importantly, when you find your true purpose in life, your work becomes something enjoyable that you're happy to do every day. There's no better feeling than knowing what you want to accomplish and recognizing how your efforts will make life better for other people. There's no more powerful combination than when your work and your life become united as one, and the synergy it produces can change your world!

Ready? Let's get started!

CHAPTER 1

Unhappy Workers and Employee Burnout

JANE IS THE CHIEF MEDICAL OFFICER at a large regional hospital. It's a role she's wanted since she was in college, and she worked hard to climb the corporate ladder. She began as a provider, but because of her desire to impact more people than those she saw in her clinical office, she began to work her way up through the ranks.

Now in her early 40s, she's attained a position of responsibility and prestige, with a generous compensation package, a corner office, a designated parking spot in the hospital garage, and the respect of her professional colleagues and community. Her home life, too, is what she always wanted, with a devoted spouse, two kids in school, and a nanny to help in the afternoons until she gets home from work.

If you asked her how she felt about her life, she'd say, "It's great! I'm living the dream. Couldn't be better. By the time I hit 50, I'm aiming to be a CEO and leave my footprint on the healthcare field."

When she was having lunch with her dad one afternoon — a retired manager at a company that made medical prosthetics — that's exactly what he asked her and what she replied. But her dad, who knew her better than most, sensed there was something deeper going on. He leaned in a little and said, "From the moment we sat down at this table, you've yawned half a dozen times. Are you getting enough sleep? What's going on, honey? You're not the same."

"C'mon, I'm fine, Dad," she said with a nervous laugh. "Who needs sleep? Between the kids and my job, I'm lucky to get five or six hours a night. And at the hospital, my boss is always talking about how he sleeps four hours a night and how anyone who requires more than that is a slacker."

Her dad looked her straight in the eye. "I'm only going to say this once: I don't know your boss, but he's either telling a tall tale to impress you, or he's headed for an early grave. Chronic sleep deprivation is no joke. Are you happy with your lifestyle?"

Jane shrugged. "To be honest, at work, we're all in the same boat. We're expected to attend breakfast meetings at 7:30 in the morning, and when we leave at 6 in the evening, we need to keep our phones handy in case we get a text or email from the overnight manager. I'll admit it's a little bit stressful. I wish I could shut off my phone when I get home."

"How about your husband, Peter?" Dad asked.

"He's fine, I think. The kids have all sorts of activities — recitals, sports games, theater — and I'm sure that keeps him very busy!"

"Sweetie, you also need to be present at these activities, don't you?"

"Of course, I go when I can!" She paused to open her purse. After rummaging through it — her dad was astonished at how much stuff she carried in there — she pulled out a small bottle of acetaminophen. She opened the bottle and tapped out two tablets. Her dad watched as she took the pills with a swallow of water. Then she put the bottle back in her purse.

"Got a headache?" he asked.

"It's very slight," she replied with a wave of her hand. "Just some tension, I think."

"How often do you get them?"

"Oh, a few times a week. It's nothing serious."

"When did they start?"

"I don't remember. Really, Dad, it's not a big deal. I survived getting COVID, didn't I? I got the vaccines just like you told me. Two shots and two boosters. I like to say I'm vaxed to the max!"

"Yes, and those shots made a huge difference to your well-being. I remember when you told me you tested positive. You spent one or two days in bed, and within a week, you went back to work."

"I would have liked to have stayed out a few more days," Jane said, "but my boss is one of *those*. If you're feeling ill, he doesn't want to hear about it. He insists he never got COVID or gets sick, but there was a week when he looked and sounded pretty awful.

To be honest, I have a feeling I got it from him, because I got sick the next week."

"The more you talk about it," her dad said, "the more it sounds like your work environment is a real pressure cooker. Are you really happy there?"

"Happy? I don't think much about being happy. Who's supposed to be happy at work?"

"*You* are."

"Really, Dad, things are a lot different than when you were working at the medical prosthetics company."

"Yes, they were different. At five o'clock, you walked out the door and went home. Managers stayed later, but not much. Every year you got your two weeks' vacation. No one took their work home with them. And the work was very satisfying, because every time we helped save someone's life by getting them the device they needed, we — all of us — could point to it and say, 'We helped that person.' Let me ask you a question: If you could change anything about your job, would you?"

"Of course, I would change many things! Sometimes I have to drag myself to work. Most mornings, when I'm sitting in my car during rush hour, listening to a motivational podcast, I feel like I want to get off the highway and keep driving until I'm far out in the country where I can hear myself think."

"You listen to motivational lectures in your car on the way to work?"

"Yes. They get me revved up to face the day."

"That and your double espresso coffee."

"Well, I need my java to get going." Jane glanced at her phone. "Oh my gosh! I've got a meeting in 15 minutes. I know it's a complete waste of time; we never accomplish anything useful in these endless meetings, but I've got to make an appearance. Love you, Daddy."

She got up, gathered her things, and hurried away from the table. With a sigh, her dad handed the server his credit card. He didn't want to say it, but he thought his daughter was heading for a bad case of burnout.

THE CREEPING MALAISE

Across America and the healthcare industry, employee burnout is emerging as a challenge to be reckoned with.

Employee burnout is defined as a state of mental, physical, and emotional exhaustion brought on by one's experiences in the workplace. If you're suffering from burnout on the job, you have difficulty engaging in activities you once found meaningful. You may no longer care about the things that are important to you, and you may experience an increasing sense of hopelessness. You feel like you're juggling as many balls as you can handle, and then life adds another ball and another until you start dropping them.

Burnout on the job is caused by excessive and prolonged stress in an environment that may once have been attractive. Burnout doesn't happen overnight; it creeps up on you, just like it's creeping up on Jane. At first, the signs and symptoms are subtle, but over time they become worse. As the stress continues, you begin to lose the interest and motivation that led you to take on a certain role.

When Jane was first hired by the hospital, she was overjoyed. It seemed like a dream job with a cutting-edge facility. She soon discovered the competitive culture was palpable. Her boss encouraged the employees to score at the top in various key performance metrics, including Leapfrog, CMS Star Ratings, and, of course, patient satisfaction! The winners were celebrated while the also-rans were made to feel like losers. It almost seemed as though her boss was trying to emulate "Neutron Jack" Welch, the CEO of GE in the 1980s who pursued the so-called "rank and yank" employment policy. Each year, Welch would fire the bottom 10% of his managers while rewarding those in the top 20% with bonuses and employee stock options.

Over time, Jane found herself increasingly dreading going to work. She felt exhausted and she got sick more often. The headaches started, and her family noticed that when she got home, she was tense and would snap at them for no apparent reason. "You guys don't *understand*," she would say. "Business is tough. You do what you have to do."

Her husband went so far as to suggest that Jane was suffering from a form of Stockholm syndrome. This condition got its name from a 1973 bank robbery in Stockholm, Sweden, in which the criminals held a group of bank employees hostage for six days. After they were set free, some of the employees refused to testify against the bank robbers in court and even raised money for their defense. As a coping mechanism, these employees had developed an affinity with their captors and had lost the ability to view their situation objectively. So it was with Jane. She was so committed to succeeding in the toxic environment of her workplace that she had lost the ability to recognize what it was doing to her.

A GLOBAL BURNOUT EPIDEMIC

Ever since the dawn of history, humans have toiled under difficult conditions. Farming and harvesting were not easy tasks. Enduring sea voyages of months or even years was dangerous. Working in tanneries or iron production was hazardous. When the Industrial Revolution swept the Western world, conditions in factories were horrendous, with children being compelled to work in textile mills for 12 hours or more a day.

But in the years after World War II, the labor conditions in the United States improved for both blue-collar and white-collar workers, and a person with a high school diploma could make enough money to buy a modest house and live comfortably. It's hard to imagine, but from its founding in 1911 until 1993, the tech giant IBM had an ironclad policy: If you did your job, you would never be laid off.

The founders of the company, Thomas Watson Sr. and his son, Thomas Watson Jr., believed that people were most productive when they felt secure. They called this value "respect for the individual," and with it came one of the most astonishing policies in American business: employment "from the cradle to the grave."

For more than seven decades, IBM never laid off a worker. If business conditions changed, workers were moved to another location, even across the country. Thus was born the IBM internal declaration, "I've Been Moved." But the company was true to its employees, and in return, they were committed to the company.

Toward the end of the 20th century, global competition intensified, and many companies, like GE under Neutron Jack, began to squeeze more productivity out of their workers. Company loyalty to their employees declined. In every industry, workers at all levels found themselves being treated like just another cost center, and corporations were determined to keep costs low and productivity high.

As the world became more competitive and companies began putting shareholder value above all else, IBM was forced to a day of reckoning. In 1993, CEO Louis V. Gerstner did the unthinkable: He approved the layoff of 60,000 workers. It was the last nail in the coffin of lifetime employment anywhere.

In some countries, the pressure on employees became unbearable. In postwar Japan, stories began to circulate of middle-aged businessmen who worked so many hours they would drop dead from stress and exhaustion or choose to end their lives rather than return to the office. The syndrome earned a name: *karoshi*, which means "overwork death." Workers who commit suicide due to mental stress are called *karōjisatsu*.

In China, the analogous "death by overwork" concept is *guolaosi*. In South Korea, it's called *gwarosa*.

In 1988, the Japanese government's Labor Force Survey reported that almost one-quarter of all male employees worked more than 60 hours per week, which, if you consider a six-day workweek, would be 10 hours per day. This is 50% longer than a typical 40-hour weekly working schedule.

In that same year, the government established the Karoshi Hotline. The hotline administrators quickly discovered that most of the people who called were not workers, but the wives of men who had either died from *karoshi* or were at high risk of doing so. This suggested that the men under workplace stress did not realize the source of their pain, were engaged in self-denial, or were under pressure to keep up the pace and not seek help.

How about healthcare workers? Up until the mid-20th century, the situation for them was different. While doctors and nurses working on the front lines of war or epidemics have always led stressful lives, the industry as a whole was highly *decentralized*. In what was still a largely agrarian economy, most doctors and nurses were self-employed in private practice. The old image of Marcus Welby, MD, the TV doctor whose show aired from 1969 to 1976, is what many Americans still remember: He was the family doctor who served the small community of Santa Monica, California, and knew all his patients personally.

I think it's safe to say that no matter what industry you're in, if you own your own business, which you control for better or worse, then your susceptibility to stress and burnout is less than if you're working for an employer who has the right and the ability to manage your time and labor. In your own practice, it's much easier to be as relaxed and easygoing as Dr. Marcus Welby!

Since the mid-20th century, the number of physicians who are self-employed in private practice has been steadily declining, and in 2020, for the first time, the percentage of self-employed doctors fell below 50%. The American Medical Association reported, "As the number of physicians in private practice has fallen, the share of physicians who work directly for a hospital or for a practice at least partially owned by a hospital or health system has increased, changing from 29.0% in 2012 to 39.8% in 2020."[1]

In the past 50 years, the healthcare industry has fallen into the familiar pattern of consolidation and growth of mega-corporations. The very first large healthcare conglomerate was the Hospital Corporation of America, founded in 1968 in Nashville, Tennessee. The three partners envisioned a company that would bring together independent hospitals to cut costs and streamline patient care — that is, to basically run a chain of hospitals like any other service business with multiple locations.

The company started with Nashville's Park View Hospital and quickly grew by acquisitions. By the end of 1981, HCA operated 349 hospitals with more than 49,000 beds. In 1992, the company went public, which meant that it faced the same shareholder pressure as any other publicly held company.

In the 2019 *Fortune 500* list of the largest United States corporations by total revenue, the company was ranked Number 67.

Today, the HCA network includes 186 hospitals and approximately 2,000 other sites of care located in 21 U.S. states and the United Kingdom. In 2022, its revenues were $60.23 billion, and it had 235,000 employees.

Perhaps, not unlike many large corporations, over the years, HCA has had its share of bad press about ethics and its treatment of its employees. In particular, HCA came under fire during the COVID-19 pandemic. As *The New York Times* reported in June 2020, despite the fact that HCA had received about $1 billion in pandemic bailout funds from the federal government, employees at HCA repeatedly complained that the company was not providing adequate personal protective equipment (PPE) to medical technicians, nurses, and cleaning staff.

The company was also in the news because of the deaths of two nurses who worked in HCA hospitals, Celia Yap-Banago in April and Rosa Luna in May, in Kansas City and California, respectively. Despite the alarm having been sounded about the lack of personal protective equipment (PPE) at work, they both contracted and died of coronavirus.[2]

By October 2021, medical workers at 19 different HCA hospitals had filed complaints with the Occupational Safety and Health Administration (OSHA) about the lack of respirator masks and being forced to reuse medical gowns.

Meanwhile, HCA executives warned that they would lay off thousands of nurses if they didn't agree to wage freezes and other concessions.[3]

The negative reports continued. As *The Independent* reported in February 2022, cleaners at HCA's London Bridge Hospital demanded a living wage, fair treatment, provision of PPE, and an end to the culture of bullying and overwork at the hospital.[4]

Physicians at HCA Bayonet Point charged that cost-cutting by HCA executives made the hospital an unsafe environment for patients, citing excessive "near misses" among patients about to undergo surgery, a slashing in the number of full-time anesthesiologists from 15 to just one, and even unsanitary conditions, including cockroaches in the operating room.[5]

The stories went on and on. For over 30 years, HCA has been the target of a steady stream of charges that it has abused employees. It's not alone; to be sure, other hospital chains have faced similar charges.

I'm shining a spotlight on this problem for two reasons: to commiserate with front-line healthcare workers and to recognize that, in addition to the challenges of providing professional care in the best environments, the job becomes exponentially more difficult — even dangerous — when the corporate employer behaves like the owner of a 19th-century sweatshop or factory.

During the pandemic, employee stress skyrocketed everywhere, and no industry was hit harder than healthcare. As *Shift Nursing* reported, during the height of the pandemic, more than one-third of nurses experienced some form of anxiety, stress, depression, and sleep disruption. A 2021 survey by the American Nurses Foundation (ANF) found that 81% of the 22,000 nurses aged 34 years and younger expressed exhaustion, 71% felt overwhelmed, and 65% reported anxiety. In 2021, 66% of critical-care nurses considered leaving the profession due to the pandemic alone.[6]

Kate Judge, executive director of the ANF, commented, "Nurses' sustained exhaustion, stress, and depression is a hit to their overall well-being and also takes a toll on our health system. This is especially so when you look at the disproportionate impact the pandemic is having on nurses who are early in their careers. As the future of our nursing profession, it is critical we give Millennials and Gen Z nurses the tools and time to recover and rebuild."[7]

Nurses who were younger had less seniority, less experience, and fewer tools with which to cope with the sudden pressures of long hours, risk to their own health, and the high rate of death they saw every day. In fact, many nurses developed post-traumatic stress disorder (PTSD), a condition found most often in soldiers serving in combat. As reported by the American Nurses Association, an integrative review by Schuster and Dwyer found that during the peak of the pandemic, about 96% of nurses reported having one or more symptoms of PTSD, with around 21% meeting the diagnostic criteria for the condition.[8]

Across the healthcare industry, employee burnout is a serious problem, and its causes are complex.

CHAPTER 2

The Two Sources of Burnout

WE KNOW THAT EMPLOYEE BURNOUT is a growing concern. You may even suffer from it yourself, or a member of your family might. No one likes it, and anyone who has it would want it to disappear. The first step in becoming free of this pernicious scourge is to understand where it comes from and the factors that contribute to it.

There are two sources of employee burnout.

The first source is your workplace.

The second source — and this may surprise you — is *you*.

No, we're not engaging in blaming the victim. If your workplace is truly toxic — racist, sexist, chaotic, corrupt, whatever — you, as an employee, may have little power to influence the behavior of your employer or manager. You can try to be a change agent, and there are examples of employees who made a difference in the culture of their workplace, sometimes by taking the company to court, but the focus of this book is squarely on what *you* can do to create a happy, productive, and fulfilling workplace for yourself.

We hear a lot of talk these days about the "work/life balance." The concept suggests that "work" and "life" are somehow two different things that sit opposed to each other on a set of scales. They may be of the same weight, but they never touch. You go to work not necessarily because you *want* to or you *like* it; you go to work because you need to make money to pay for your life: your house, your boat, your club membership. Of course, it's nice if you enjoy your work, but the gap between the two is wide. You need a "balance" because if you have too much work, you need to offset it with a better life. Work itself cannot make you happy in your life.

In our wealthy, industrialized society, most of us have a choice as to what we can do to support ourselves. Few of us are forced to work at a job just because it's the only one available. This element of choice gives you, the potential employee, some quantum of power in the employment marketplace. If your workplace is truly horrendous, or if you're employed in an industry that you simply don't like, then you owe it to yourself to vote with your feet and find a vocation that you can commit to.

In the pages ahead, we'll talk much more about breaking down the artificial barrier between "work" and "life" and the desirability of creating what I call a *work/life synergy*. This is where, instead of sitting on opposite ends of a set of scales, never touching, your work and your life have a close relationship, and the artificially contrived gap between the two is closed. In other words, there is no scale, just one weight composed of "work" and "life."

It's not all doom and gloom, and statistically, doctors often have long careers with a good work/life synergy. As of 2023, the oldest practicing physician on record was Howard Tucker, MD, a neurologist in Cleveland, Ohio. At more than 100 years old, he had been practicing medicine since 1947. He stopped seeing patients, but he was still training medical residents and doing medical review work from his home. His 75 years of practice were memorialized in the *Guinness Book of World Records*.

His wife of 65 years, Sara Tucker, was a psychiatrist who still practiced psychoanalysis at age 89.

Dr. Tucker told Psychiatrist.com, "I thoroughly enjoy teaching my medical residents and students, and I learn a great deal from them as well. It's been a joy to share stories from my long career with the next generation."[9]

The work/life synergy of human beings can be exceedingly complex, which is why we're going to take it step by step and avoid generalizations. In this chapter, we're going to proceed on the assumption that you want to stay in your current healthcare role, but you also want to avoid getting burned out. To do that and to spare yourself the fate that's slowly creeping up on Jane, who doesn't realize she's suffering from burnout, you should know the root causes of the malady: Is it your workplace, your home life, or a combination of the two?

YOUR STRESSFUL WORKPLACE

When you do the same boring thing every day, you're going to get burned out. And yes, this even applies to people on the front lines of healthcare who, according to the stereotype established by society, are supposed to be deeply grateful to have the opportunity to heal people and save lives. They should be happy to work long hours under stressful conditions with low pay, all because they're doing a special job that brings its own unique rewards.

Let's get that myth out of the way. It's true that healthcare workers in every job position should feel a particular satisfaction that people in other industries may not enjoy, but that's no excuse for oppressive work conditions, low pay, and high rates of burnout. The lives of healthcare workers, from the top executive to the entry-level orderly, are just as valuable as any others.

For any worker, the source of burnout could be their work, or it could be the opposite: *not* having work. Some people are overworked and have burnout, while others are underworked and experience the same fate.

There are people who spend many hours at work, and their family members long for them to be at home. There are other situations where they may be at home, and their family hopes they find a job and get out of the house! This is a big problem for retirees, which we'll talk about in the pages ahead. People who work simply to retire often find themselves with a big problem: They're bored. They need a new goal and a new challenge.

You've heard the expression "TGIF" or "Thank God It's Friday." We even have a restaurant chain named after it. It means we're living for the weekend; in other words, we endure the work week so we can enjoy the relaxing weekend. That's unfortunate and could be interpreted to mean that many people are doing work that doesn't mean too much to them except for getting a paycheck to earn a living.

If the work we do at our job does not add some meaning to our lives, then we shouldn't be doing it.

For most people who suffer from burnout, the most significant source is their workplace. But that word is very general, and at their workplace, there's usually not just one source of burnout but several. When you look closely, the debilitating effects are often an aggregation of many problem areas, some of which can be fixed. In the workplace, contributors to burnout can include the following:

Having Little or No Control Over Your Work

If you feel like a cog in the machine, carrying out orders and directions from your manager with no input into how you do your job, you'll quickly become bored. You'll act like the nurse who rooms a patient, offers no smile and no conversation, and just tells the hapless victim to take a seat and the doctor will be in shortly before walking out and slamming the door.

This can be a function of the variety in your role. You might assume that if your job requires many repetitive tasks, such as assembly line work, it will be boring. Yes, it might be tedious, but under the right circumstances, it can be interesting. Within most organizations controlled by rational people, the leaders are smart enough to know that front-line employees are a potent source of new ideas for innovation and improvement. Who better to detect flaws in the system and suggest improvements than someone deeply involved in that system?

To keep employees engaged while leveraging their talents and experience, many corporations, including those in the healthcare industry, have *hackathons*, which are brainstorming events in which employees at all levels are turned loose to explore and develop innovative ideas that can improve the product or service.

For example, in October 2022, Johnson & Johnson Nursing launched its first NurseHack4Health Pitch-A-Thon, a weekend event in which 10 nurse-led multidisciplinary health system teams were invited to pitch their solutions for redesigning a healthcare workplace where nurses and other healthcare professionals can thrive.

Over the course of the weekend of this nationwide virtual event, nurse hackers worked together to propose and develop solutions that included a mental health platform for adolescents that leverages gamification, a universal way to report health-related misinformation, and an app that can share accurate and real-time vaccine information.[10]

These nurses don't feel like robots. They know they're helping to improve healthcare for all of us.

Take some time and ask yourself some questions: Do you see areas of the systems you use at work that could be improved? When you have an idea, does your manager listen to you? Or do they brush you off and tell you to get back to work?

Lack of Recognition

No one likes to toil in obscurity, especially in an organization where job success can have tangible rewards, such as promotions and pay raises. Employees who lack positive feedback from their boss and colleagues may begin to wonder whether their work makes any difference. Such employees will be tempted to "quietly quit," which means they just coast along, doing the absolute minimum necessary to collect their paycheck. Many jobs in healthcare are overlooked or underappreciated. For example, registration staff are crucial for setting the tone of the visit, dealing with angry patients, and managing expectations, but they are rarely praised when things are running smoothly due in part to their contributions.

Some managers believe that the time and place to deliver praise is the annual employee review. That's crazy! By that time, it's too late. Managers need to practice a policy of offering quick public praise at the time of the action or result. It needn't be a big production — just saying, "Hey, Jane, your report on the campaign was very good. Thank you!" is all you need.

Ask yourself: How often do you have positive personal contact with your manager? Do you feel as though your efforts are recognized? Or do you think if you "quietly quit," no one would notice?

Lofty Goal Setting / Performance Expectations

Sometimes managers thoughtlessly assign work that people simply cannot accomplish or set goals that are far out of reach. A classic case emerged in 2016 when Wells Fargo was accused of forcing its employees to meet impossible sales goals. To meet those goals, bank employees fraudulently signed up customers for credit cards and other products they had not requested. Between 2011 and 2016, the number of unauthorized deposit accounts and credit card accounts opened for unwitting customers reached a staggering 3.5 million.

As the story broke in the national news and Wells Fargo paid substantial fines, CEO John Stumpf dodged responsibility and blamed faulty sales practices rather than the corrupt company culture.

Employees at Wells Fargo reported extreme feelings of burnout. Under intense pressure to sell, many described levels of stress that led to crying, vomiting, and severe panic attacks. To cope with the pressure, at least one employee secretly consumed hand sanitizer that contained alcohol. Some reported that calls to the company's ethics hotline were met with either no reaction or resulted in the employee making the call being fired. One bank employee told NPR, "We were all miserable, and it was just soul crushing to walk in every day."[11]

This is reminiscent of the situation in many large pharmacy chains that impose profit-driven sales quotas, such as filling a minimum number of prescriptions per hour or enrolling 40% of patients into automatic refill programs, which have nothing to do with the safe practice of medicine. They give pharmacists a range of metrics to meet, and they monitor the time spent on various tasks, from prescriptions filled and vaccinations given per day to the number and duration of calls to patients. Pharmacists say the chains began to push them harder when profit margins began to shrink after the Great Recession.

"Basically, your day is timed out by the minute," an Alabama pharmacist told NBC News. "It's like the worst case of micromanaging you can imagine."[12]

Ask yourself: Does your manager consult you about your workload, or simply tell you what to do? Do you feel as though your company sets realistic goals and helps you attain them? Or are you under extreme pressure to deliver results you know are out of reach?

Monotonous or Unchallenging Work

Life is changing, and the rate of technological progress is increasing every day. As human beings, we thrive on challenges and the opportunity to grow and take on new responsibilities. That's why it can be dispiriting to have a job that's the same, day in and day out. There's only one cure for this condition: You either need to move up the organizational ladder or take on additional tasks that allow you to flex different skillsets, which will sharpen your mind and keep that bounce in your step as you walk into work each day. You need a job that is stimulating and challenging enough that you enjoy doing it every day.

Ask yourself: At your work, are you challenged and compelled to keep learning? If your work is repetitive, do you have the opportunity to cross-train and tackle other roles? Or are you coasting, stuck in a rut, doing the same thing every day?

Chaotic Environment

Humans like having clear goals and a path toward achieving those goals. While an element of risk at work is healthy and exciting, few of us enjoy working in an environment that's completely chaotic and directionless. A chaotic workplace is evident in "spinning your wheels," where people seem super-busy all day, every day, but they're doing tasks that don't move the organization forward. They're constantly putting out fires and urgently responding to imaginary crises. Because people are intently focused on today's tasks, real long-term improvements are rare.

A chaotic workplace could also include duplicating work or considering everything a "top" priority. One of the hallmarks of a well-run organization is that leadership establishes clear goals then helps the employees break down each goal into smaller, prioritized sections or sprints. Every workday, you should be assigned a focused goal and be empowered to decide how you're going to allocate your time to deliver the most important results. Everything you're asked to do should help the company fulfill its mission and meet a stated objective.

Leaders must properly allocate the labor available to avoid needless duplication, turf battles, or competition among employees. Teams are vital to any business, but every team needs a coach to keep the group focused and productive!

Ask yourself: Is there a sustained effort in your workplace to achieve a clearly articulated common goal? Or are people running around in a frenzy, expending much energy but accomplishing little? And do you feel as though you can go to your manager and say, "I have several tasks on my desk. Please prioritize them for me. Which one do you want completed first?"

Toxic Culture

Sadly, some toxic work environments are characterized by co-workers and managers who are more interested in tearing down or intimidating their colleagues than working with them for the common good. Personal intrusions into your space can include acts of racism, sexism, jealousy, passive-aggressive behavior, negativity, invitations to engage in unethical activity — you name it!

The fact is, company culture begins at the top and trickles down. For example, in 2018, *The New York Times* revealed that four years earlier, tech giant Google, which had long been accused of having a work environment toxic to women and minorities, had handed Andy Rubin, the creator of Android mobile software, an astonishing $90 million exit package. What Google did not announce was that an employee had accused Rubin of sexual misconduct. Google had investigated and concluded her claim was credible, and Rubin was secretly asked to leave the company. Instead of treating Rubin like royalty, Google could have fired him and paid him little to nothing as the door slammed behind him.

Rubin was one of three executives that Google allegedly protected over the past decade after they were accused of sexual misconduct. Shortly after the revelation by the *Times*, thousands of Google employees in cities around the world — including Singapore, Hyderabad (India), Berlin, Zurich, London, Chicago, and Seattle — held a wave of walkouts to protest the tech company's handling of sexual harassment.[13]

We usually think of a toxic culture as one under which an employee must suffer because of a thoughtless leader at the top. Once in a while, however, the *leader* is the one who unwittingly creates the toxic culture, recognizes it and takes radical action to remake it into something good and uplifting.

Here's a real-world example of someone who did exactly that — and it opened the door to success he never imagined.

In 1989, Brian Scudamore was a 19-year-old high school dropout in Vancouver, Canada. He had dreams of going to college, but he had no money. One day, while waiting in the drive-through lane of a McDonald's restaurant, Scudamore happened to see an old, beat-up pickup truck emblazoned with the words "Mark's Hauling." The truck was for a trash removal company.

"I can do that!" Scudamore thought.

Scudamore then spent $700 on an old Ford F-100 pickup truck and another $300 on fliers and business cards. It was his entire life savings. (His parents were extremely annoyed he had dropped out of high school and told him he needed to pay his own way.) Even though the business was a one-man operation, he called it The Rubbish Boys. "I wanted it to sound bigger," he told *CNBC Make It.*

In a few weeks, Scudamore had made back his investment. After a year, he had made a profit of about $1,700, which he used to cover his college tuition.[14]

But as the fledgling business grew, he faced a new challenge: *his own burnout.*

As he told Bench.co, by 1994, he had been running his business for five years and was earning half a million in revenues. But he no longer enjoyed the work. Why not? Because, as the boss, he felt like he was spending his day listening to his 11 employees complain. They griped about the job, about the weather, about having to work late, about not making enough money. To avoid interacting with them, Scudamore began to hide in his office. He'd hand out the paperwork in the morning and then close his door, which almost certainly made the employees' attitudes even worse.

One day, he came to a momentous decision. He realized that he had created the negative culture in his company by hiring the wrong people. He had tried to hire people who he thought had the right skills, but that had been a big mistake. There was only one way to solve the problem: fire everyone and start over from the ground up.

That's exactly what he did. He got them together and said, "Guys, I've let you down. I haven't found the right people or given you the love and support you need to be successful. I'm the one that messed up here, I've made a big mistake, and my sincerest apologies, but I'm letting everyone go."[15]

He went back to ground zero with just himself and one truck. He vowed only to hire people who had a positive attitude — or as he said, "Optimists who will see problems as opportunities versus just challenges that they need to fight through." He wanted guys with whom he could hang out. Their skill level didn't matter; he could teach them what they needed to know.

It was extremely difficult, but he stuck to his plan. He hired very carefully, and after six months, he was back where he had been, but now he was poised to expand the business through a franchise model.

In 1997, the business hit $1 million in annual revenue.

Today, the business, which in 1999 Scudamore renamed 1-800-GOT-JUNK?, operates junk-removal franchises in roughly 160 locations in the U.S., Canada, and Australia. Valued at over $300 million, it's the main component of a bigger family of brands launched by Scudamore that includes a house-painting company, WOW 1 Day Painting, and a home-detailing business, Shack Shine, which Scudamore founded in 2010 and 2015, respectively.

"Did I know that day that this would be something much bigger than just a way to pay for college? No," Scudamore said. "But I knew that if I picked something and I committed and stuck with it, the passion for building a business would soon follow."

On Glassdoor, the site where employees rate their own company and their CEO, 1-800-GOT-JUNK? scores a respectable 3.4 stars out of five. In January 2023, 63% of employees said they'd recommend it to a friend who was looking for a job. Fifty-seven percent said the company had a positive business outlook, and an impressive 72% expressed approval for CEO Brian Scudamore.[16]

Ask yourself: Does your company offer a healthy, supportive work environment? Is there true inclusiveness? (Not just diversity; they are two different things. You can have plenty of diversity with little inclusiveness!) Or do you feel the sting of discrimination from one or more of your colleagues? Do you see certain employees or managers getting preferential treatment from leaders?

If you're the owner or CEO, do you love coming to work every day? Do you have a positive and uplifting spirit, or are you locked in your office because you don't want to interact with your own employees? If it's your company, you can change the culture!

YOUR OWN LIFESTYLE

While you may have limited control over your workplace environment, you have significant control over your own lifestyle. Here are some of the factors that can contribute to burnout if you allow them to persist.

All Work and No Play

Everyone needs a break from their work, even if they love it and don't regard it as drudgery. For example, consider Warren Buffett. An occasional owner of the title "World's Wealthiest Person," Buffett has been working at his career as a professional investor for his entire adult life. He has never retired, and at age 92, he still goes to his office in Omaha, Nebraska, six days a week. His work ethic has been described as relentless, but if you dig deeper, you see how he avoids burnout.

- He sleeps a solid eight hours a night in his own modest home.
- He avoids scheduling meetings in advance. As Bill Gates wrote, "One habit of Warren's that I admire is that he keeps his schedule free of meetings. He's good at saying 'no' to things. He knows what he likes to do — and what he does, he does unbelievably well."[17]
- He loves to play bridge. "I play a lot," Buffett told Thomas Heath of the *Washington Post* in a 2017 interview. "At least four sessions a week, about two hours a session." That's at least eight hours a week.[18]
- He plays a mean ukulele. Buffett picked up the instrument when he was 18 (he was trying to impress a girl) and has never stopped playing. In a 2013 interview with the *Omaha World-Herald*, Hawaiian ukulele virtuoso Jake Shimabukuro said, "[Warren is] a serious player, man. He knows his chords and he knows his tunes." Referring to Warren Buffett and Bill Gates (who plays one too), he said, "It blows my mind that

these people, who have everything in the world they could want, have picked up the ukulele and found a little bit of joy."[19]

When Warren Buffet is at the office, he focuses intently on work, but you can be sure that when he's playing bridge or the ukulele, he's *not* thinking about work.

One personal habit of Buffett's that you should *not* emulate is his diet. He literally subsists on Coca-Cola, cookies, ice cream, and McDonald's fast food — breakfast, lunch, and dinner. Please do not do this! For most people, such a diet can lead to malnutrition, obesity, heart disease, and diabetes. (Yes, you can suffer from both malnutrition *and* obesity. Obesity is often characterized by a paradoxical state of malnutrition, which, despite excessive energy consumption, is associated with a lack of individual micronutrients.)

Ask yourself: Does your career give you enough time and space to get away from work *every day*? Or, like Jane, do you feel chained to your job from morning 'til night? And on a deeper level, do you regard your work as a necessary hardship you must endure to earn a paycheck, or as something you'd like to do even if you weren't paid?

As Warren Buffett said in a 1998 speech at the University of Florida, "There comes a time when you ought to start doing what you want. Take a job that you love. You will jump out of bed in the morning.... You really should take a job that if you were independently wealthy, that would be the job you would take."[20]

Lack of Close, Supportive Relationships

Humans are, by nature, social animals. Since the days of the cave men, we've learned that our survival is enhanced by forming close social bonds and supporting each other. Numerous studies have shown that people with strong social relationships — not necessarily marriage *per se* — live longer than those who don't. For example, a meta-analytic review by researchers Julianne Holt-Lunstad, Timothy B. Smith, and J. Bradley Layton found that "the influence of social relationships on the risk of death are comparable with well-established risk factors for mortality such as smoking and alcohol consumption and exceed the influence of other risk factors such as physical inactivity and obesity."[21]

Ask yourself: Both at work and at home, do you have friends and loved ones who provide support and who need your support in return? Or do you go home alone and sit in front of the television or stare at your phone?

Biting Off More Than You Can Chew

It's up to you to control your workload, even if it means going to your boss and saying, "I cannot perform all these tasks myself. Please either prioritize them for me or ask another team member to take some of the load."

Accepting too many responsibilities is also a big problem with entrepreneurs who, as their company grows, are either reluctant to give up the tasks they've always done or don't trust anyone else to do them. Plus, digital devices make it easier to work remotely, but they also make it possible to work all the time. As your weekly work hours increase, so do your feelings of pressure and stress.

Ask yourself: At work, do you have confidence that if you took a few sick days, your colleagues could pick up the slack? Or do you feel you need to be there all day, every day, just to keep up?

Not Enough Sleep

Like Jane, you may suffer from sleep deprivation and not realize it. (If you have a new baby in the house, then you can skip to the next item! You'll get more sleep as your little angel gets older.) The sad fact is that many Americans are sleep-deprived. According to the American Sleep Apnea Association, 70% of adults report that they get insufficient sleep at least one night a month, and 11% report getting insufficient sleep *every* night. It's estimated that sleep-related problems affect 50 to 70 million Americans of all ages and socio-economic classes.

And the trends are going in the wrong direction. As the lines between work and home have become blurred and digital technology has become entrenched in our lives, the odds of being sleep deprived (getting fewer than six hours of sleep a night) have increased significantly over the past 30 years. The National Institutes of Health predicts that America's "sleep debt" is rising, and that by the middle of the 21st century, more than 100 million Americans will have difficulty falling asleep.[22]

Contrary to the boasts of Jane's boss, sleep deprivation comes at a high price. While work stress and schedules can affect your ability to get good sleep, the opposite is true, too. If you've ever dozed off at your desk or during an important meeting, you know that sleep deprivation can greatly reduce your work performance. It can leave you feeling exhausted and bleary-eyed and make it more difficult to stay focused on important projects.

Sleep deprivation is a symptom *of shift work disorder*, which affects people who work night, early morning, and rotating shifts. The disorder may cause insomnia when night workers attempt to sleep in the daytime, as well as extreme sleepiness while they are at work. The average person with shift work disorder loses one to four hours of sleep per night.

Outside of work, drowsy driving or simply falling asleep at the wheel is a factor in up to 20% of all serious motor vehicle crash injuries.[23] While driving, have you ever experienced microsleep? You probably have without even knowing it. Researchers define microsleep as sleep episodes that last for 15 seconds or less. During a microsleep episode, you're literally driving blind. Your eyes may remain open, but key parts of your brain have turned off.

Try to remember that sleep is a necessary part of the proper functioning of the human brain. It's not a "luxury" that lazy people indulge in. It's not wasted time. While you sleep, your brain is busy processing the day's events and preparing for tomorrow.

Ask yourself: Does your job allow you to go home and get an adequate night's sleep? Some transportation industries, particularly airlines and trucking, have regulations limiting the length of time an employee can be on duty, but most have no such restrictions. When you go home, can you disconnect from work and not have to answer any texts or emails? And even if you can disconnect from work, do you voluntarily unplug from all electronics an hour before bedtime?

Perfectionistic Tendencies

This is a tricky one. In some occupations, such as brain surgery and manned space flight, you and everyone on your team need to strive for perfection. There can be no mistakes. If this is the case with you, then another requirement is that you must have the resources to do your job properly. If perfection is the goal, then it must be an organizational priority.

For example, consider the tragic explosion and destruction of the space shuttle *Challenger* on January 26, 1986. The cause was traced to faulty O-rings in the solid rocket boosters, which in the freezing weather that morning, had failed. The real tragedy is that many of the engineers at Morton Thiokol, which built the boosters, knew about the problem and raised red flags about it, but they were overruled by project managers. In that case, a little *more* perfectionism could have saved the craft and crew from disaster.

But in normal life, an unreasonable drive toward perfection can be a big problem. Such an obsession has its roots in an exaggerated fear of failure. In the logic of the perfectionist, if the project or product is *not yet perfect*, then it cannot be released, therefore saving the team from the possibility of failure.

This human tendency to avoid the exposure of imperfection has been largely conquered in the software industry, which, if you follow agile methodology, has embraced imperfection as a practical way to keep a project moving forward. It's assumed that each new iteration of a piece of software is imperfect and that its flaws will be revealed through real-world use and corrected in the next iteration. This is a fitting example of the axiom "Perfect is the enemy of the good." Attributed to Voltaire, it's a reflection of the fact that achieving absolute perfection is impossible, and so, as increasing the investment or effort results in diminishing returns, further activity becomes increasingly inefficient and pointless.

There's a similar ancient Chinese saying: "Better a diamond with a flaw than a pebble without one." It means you should consider the overall value of your endeavor or product, not just its level of perfection.

There is a difference between the pursuit of perfection and the pursuit of excellence. Perfection is an unattainable dream, while excellence is an attribute that everyone can strive for. This is particularly true in healthcare, where we're trying to maintain a machine — the human body and brain — that is far more complex than we can understand! In such a dynamic and nuanced environment, perfection is impossible, and instead, clinicians must rely on time-tested values and standards by which to judge their work. Often, the only metrics healthcare providers can use is, "Have we been able to relieve their pain and suffering? Is their disease in remission? How much time have we added to this person's happy, healthy life?"

Ask yourself: What is the reasonableness of your standard of perfection? If you manufacture 10,000 units of a product, how many defects in that product will you tolerate? If you want zero defects, what resources are you willing to commit to achieving that goal? At what point are you going to say, "We've done our very best, and we're going to move on"?

Need to Be in Control

The control freak is the close cousin of the perfectionist, but the difference relates to how a project unfolds *over time*. Let's say you're a project manager. You design a project, assemble a team, and map out the timeline to completion. What follows brings to mind the line from poet Robert Burns: "The best-laid schemes of mice and men often go awry." Indeed, they do!

There are at least two reasons why being a "control freak" is not a good strategy.

The first is that if you insist on your vision being the only one considered, you're taking the stand that you are the only authority and only your ideas matter; the viewpoints of others are not worthy of consideration. This is extremely foolish. Remember the words of Steve Jobs, who said, "It doesn't make sense to hire smart people and tell them what to do; we hire smart people so they can tell us what to do."

Surround yourself with smart people and listen to them! As your business grows, you'll find that you need subject matter experts with knowledge and experience beyond your own, just as in your personal life, you seek the services of doctors, lawyers, electricians, and plumbers to keep your life running smoothly.

Delegating authority to others whom they hire can be difficult for entrepreneurs who have a singular vision and have become accustomed to doing everything themselves. They just don't trust anyone else to care about their "baby" as much as they do. They see themselves at the helm of a ship tossing in a storm at sea, and they don't want anyone else to take the wheel.

In any business, many ubiquitous tasks can and must be delegated. The first jobs to be filled often include accounting and financial management because they are not close to the core of the business. A good accountant or finance manager could work for any company. Then you can delegate or hire for human resources and facilities management or fabrication.

You can also outsource these functions; for example, the vast majority of consumer products companies outsource the manufacturing or "co-packing" (short for "contract packing") of their products. Then, you can hire people for sales and order fulfillment. Again, these are ubiquitous jobs. Eventually, most entrepreneurs spend their valuable time overseeing the activities of their little army of people while also dealing with the *real* bosses — the investors. Ideally, your companies will grow and become self-sufficient enough that you can take on a purely supervisory role.

In healthcare, providers often form personal relationships with their patients, which can make delegating difficult. Even when a physician refers a patient to another trusted doctor, like a specialist, the primary care physician may have a hard time letting go and trusting the next doctor to take full responsibility for the consult. This is the reason trust among colleagues is so important, not only in healthcare but in every industry.

Richard Branson started in business at the age of 16 with a magazine called *Student* and, in 1970, he opened a mail-order record store. Now, more than 50 years later, he presides over a vast empire comprising more than 400 businesses in industries encompassing books, ocean cruises, space travel, hotels, media, mobile communications, music, wines, and more.

He's a smart person, but there's no way he's a genius in every one of those sectors, nor could he possibly oversee their day-to-day operations. He's the ultimate delegator, which leaves him time to pursue his various hobbies; he's an expert at kitesurfing and has set two world records in the sport, including, in 2012, being the oldest person to kitesurf across the English Channel. Other achievements range from setting the record in 1987 for the first hot air balloon to cross the Atlantic to his 1991 record of piloting the first balloon across the Pacific from Japan to Arctic Canada.

As Branson wrote in a blog post, "Most entrepreneurs are driven personalities, but you can't overcome challenges and bring new ideas to the market through the sheer force of personality alone. You need to learn to delegate so that you can focus on the big picture.... As your business grows, seek out people who understand your ideas, want to build on them, and can envision ways to make improvements in your business. As your responsibilities increase, delegating those that others can do better will free you to plan for the future and find new ways to develop your company."[24]

It's possible to create and operate a big hospital that's human-centered and values the health and well-being of its employees and partners, as does the Mayo Clinic. This renowned medical center, headquartered in Rochester, Minnesota, and operating several campuses across the United States, is known for its multidisciplinary approach, whereby doctors of different expertise are charged with the care of a patient. With 63,000 employees, it's consistently ranked among the top hospitals in the world and is known for its patient-centered care and collaborative approach to medicine.

Here are just a few of the hallmarks of the Mayo Clinic:

Team-based care: At Mayo Clinic, patient care is delivered by a team of specialists from various medical disciplines, including physicians, surgeons, nurses, therapists, and other healthcare professionals. This team-based approach ensures that patients receive comprehensive and coordinated care tailored to their specific needs.

Collaborative decision-making: Mayo Clinic emphasizes shared decision-making between patients and their healthcare teams. Patients are encouraged to actively participate in their treatment plans, and medical professionals work together to devise the most effective and personalized care strategies.

Integrated facilities: The Mayo Clinic campuses are designed to foster collaboration among medical specialists. Facilities are equipped with state-of-the-art technology and resources that support the seamless sharing of patient information and facilitate communication between different departments.

Research and innovation: Mayo Clinic's emphasis on innovation and evidence-based medicine allows it to stay at the forefront of medical advancements. This enables the hospital to offer its patients cutting-edge treatments and therapies.

Education and training: The organization is committed to education and training, and its physicians and staff regularly participate in continuing education programs. This commitment to learning ensures that the hospital's medical teams are up to date with the latest medical knowledge and best practices.

Patient-focused environment: The hospital places a strong emphasis on patient satisfaction and experience. They strive to create a welcoming and supportive environment where patients and their families feel well-informed and cared for throughout their healthcare journey.

Ask yourself: What do you really need to control, and what can you delegate to others? Is there any point to clinging to your preconceived plan, or should you be open to new ideas that you haven't considered? Isn't it better to be like the surfer who rides the wave rather than the guy who tries to swim against it?

Unreasonable Rigidity

There are two types of fatal rigidity in business: planning and personal.

Plans are necessary, and leaders make them for all sorts of reasons: to attract funding, build partnerships, anticipate future growth, or guide development. To attempt to grow without any plan or set of goals is extremely risky, but no plan is carved in stone. Every plan must be periodically reviewed and adjusted to meet current realities. This is because disruption and change are the new laws of business.

The strategic plan you design today will be challenged by seismic shifts coming at you tomorrow. The business leaders (and I hope you see yourself as a leader, if not now, then in the future) who succeed and avoid burnout are those who can roll with change and are flexible and ready to adapt. To cling to a hopelessly rigid way of doing things just because it's "in the plan" is foolish and can lead to disaster.

Personal rigidity can be a liability. In this case, we make a strong distinction between your preferences and what the real world may require. Cultural norms evolve, and you must be able to adjust to them. If you're an "old school" leader who doesn't understand the power of social media to define brands, then you need to become flexible and embrace the digital age. Your competitors are moving ahead, and in the scramble to hire and retain the very best talent, you need to stay on top.

Ask yourself: Do you have a solid business plan? Do you know where you want to be in the next five years? Have you recently reviewed you plan to ensure it's up to date with today's reality?

You have your personal values, which will never change, but are your operational methods in alignment with the competitive landscape? Is your company attracting the very best and brightest people to join your team?

Survivor's Guilt

While survivor's guilt is most acute in the healthcare industry, you also see it in the military and, more mildly, in any situation where, despite the best efforts of the team, the project has failed.

The COVID-19 pandemic brought this issue to the forefront. Across America and around the world, thousands of front-line doctors and nurses experienced feelings of guilt and inadequacy as they saw their patients die before their eyes. They then had to deliver the terrible news to the surviving family members, many of whom, in their grief, may have blamed the doctor for not doing more to save their loved one.

Survivor's guilt is a form of post-traumatic stress disorder (PTSD). It's a very simple problem: The afflicted person asks themselves, "Why am I still alive while the other person is dead or grievously injured?" Often, there is no good answer to this question other than,

"The world has no rules. Things happen at random. That's all." But human beings hate that answer. We like to believe there is a cause-and-effect relationship to every event, good or bad. Morality plays a role, too: Deep down inside, we feel that if we lead a good and ethical life, we have a better chance of avoiding bad events, and conversely, people who suffer misfortune may have invited it through their "bad karma."

Guilt can be deeply ingrained since childhood. As Lawrence D. Blum noted in *JAMA Internal Medicine*, "All sorts of experiences in childhood, such as deaths in the family, illnesses, traumas, abuse, divorce, and problematic relationships, can saddle a person with an unrecognized burden of guilt. This guilt may be hidden for a long time, but then play an important role in later years."[25]

In a meta-analysis completed *before* the COVID-19 pandemic, researchers at the Missouri State Medical Association found that "mental illness and burnout are epidemic in physicians and medical trainees. One study found 20% of medical residents met criteria for depression while 74% met criteria for burnout."[26]

It's well-known that while relative to the general population, physicians have a lower mortality risk from common causes such as cancer and heart disease, they have a higher rate of suicide than the general population. Each year in the U.S., roughly 300 to 400 physicians die by suicide, and suicide deaths are as much as 400% higher among female physicians when compared to females in other professions.

I hope you understand that many sources of career burnout are not only the things that you would immediately identify as being negative habits or practices, such as not getting enough sleep or working in a chaotic environment. There are many seemingly positive habits or practices, such as an overwhelming drive to perfection that, when taken a step too far, are equally as dangerous.

For example, think about the healthcare profession. It can be difficult for doctors and nurses to accept the fact that imperfection and failure are built-in features of the profession. Healthcare workers can help many people and save many lives, but sometimes the disease wins. Particularly during a high-stress event such as the COVID-19 pandemic, when it seemed as though the tide of death was too strong to stop, and sick and dying people languished in hospital hallways while the disease ran rampant, it's all too easy to sacrifice one's own physical and mental health in the service of others. But this is the reality: In the healthcare profession, no one can give people eternal life; death comes to us all. The job description is to prolong healthy life and delay the inevitable onset of death for as long as possible.

If you understand this, no matter what your chosen profession, the very best thing you can do for yourself and your community is to get up at sunrise with a glad heart and spend the day doing your very best work. At sunset, you put away your tools and take your well-deserved rest until tomorrow. If everyone did that, wouldn't the world be a happier place?

Ask yourself: Do you feel guilty that you enjoy health and good fortune while other people suffer? Do you accuse yourself of being selfish if you don't sacrifice yourself for others? Do you go home at night and criticize yourself for not doing more to help others?

CHAPTER 3

Finding Work/Life Synergy

WE CAN ALL AGREE THAT EMPLOYEE BURNOUT — *your* burnout — is a bad thing. It makes you miserable, affects your job performance, and may even negatively impact your mental and physical health.

If you feel burned out at work — or bored, exhausted, sleepless, disgruntled, or even angry — what can you do about it?

You can begin by asking yourself some tough questions about who you are and what you want from life. We began this process in the previous chapter, but in the pages ahead, we're going to dive more deeply into it.

Before we do that, let's think about an idea that has become popular in the past few decades: the "work/life balance." As a social and economic concept, it has its roots in the Industrial Revolution, which hit its stride in the 20th century. It's an offshoot of a school of thought called "structural functionalism," which viewed society as a body comprised of various organs, all of which performed their own tasks for the benefit of the whole.

This post-war theory asserted a radical separation between work (institution, workplace, or market) and family. Men and women conducted their activities in separate spheres, with women at home doing the "expressive work" of raising children and men in the public workplace performing "instrumental tasks" of creating goods and services.

The goal, it would seem, was efficiency, with a big dose of sexism thrown in. This was strictly an industrial age concept; people living in an agrarian culture, which the entire world was for thousands of years, would find it nonsensical. On a farm, everyone works and everyone contributes to economic production.

In any case, such a system would lead to concern about one's work/life balance, with men focused only on industrial work and women stuck at home. In the 21st century, the nature of work is changing, and the old male/female stereotypes are fading. We have more mobility and more choices, both at home and at work. We're rejecting the notion that working to earn a paycheck is something that's not supposed to be enjoyable.

In my own experience, staff and physician colleagues often ask me about their work/life balance. My initial thought and question back to them is why do we even use the phrase "work/life balance"? "Balance" implies that we are offsetting one thing with another; in this case, our work is being offset by our non-working life. This implies a confrontation between life and work. Why must this be? Why should our experience at work be so dramatically different from our experience outside of work?

The reality is that many people see work as a burden or an obstacle standing in the way of a pleasurable life. In this situation, people are going to work simply to earn a living, not because they receive true fulfillment and enjoyment. At its worst, an individual will get into a vicious cycle of working at a job they don't really like to buy stuff they don't really require in order to show off to people they don't really care about. That's a sad way to live.

The first thing we need to do is break this cycle. To do this, we must change our perspective and see work as a part of a happy, fulfilling life. It truly is a different dimension of our life. Once we appreciate and acknowledge that we are constantly living our lives regardless of location (work or outside of work), we can turn our attention to our particular job.

If you're not engaged in work that you are passionate about, then you should start asking yourself some questions. Ultimately, our time at work and outside of work should contribute to our energy, our passion, and our purpose, not detract or stand in the way of it. In other words, we must consider how we can make work and life synergistic with each other and achieve not work/life *balance* but work/life *synergy*.

In this case, synergy means the interaction of two or more areas of your life to produce a combined effect greater than the sum of their separate effects. The old saying, "The whole is greater than the sum of its parts," expresses the basic meaning of synergy.

If you're passionate about your work and it means something

to you, then you'll find that you're not only more productive at work but also more present and engaged at home, and vice versa. When you get good news at home, you'll bring that exuberance to the workplace, and that energy will become infectious to your coworkers and the projects you are working on. Achieving work/life synergy has the potential to result in your becoming more fulfilled in all aspects of life: a better husband, wife, mother, father, brother, sister, boss, coworker, friend — all the roles you play in life.

The interesting thing about synergy is that you can't achieve it unless all the constituent parts are harmonious and blend well. Not literally, perhaps, but *in your heart.*

Here's an example. Let's say Dave works at Acme Technology Corporation, a company that manufactures medical supplies — not glamorous, high-tech devices, but everyday things like exam gloves and feeding bags. At the end of the day, Dave comes home from work. At the dinner table, his partner asks, "So, how was your day?"

In one scenario, Dave replies, "Just the usual. Nothing to talk about. After all, it's just medical supplies. It's really quite boring. What's on television tonight?"

In another scenario, Dave replies, "We're designing this really cool new walker boot that's 20% lighter than the old walker boots. It's made from a new type of plastic, so when one patient is done with it, instead of just throwing it away, it can be recycled. It's designed to be especially useful in developing nations because it's cheaper to ship, and we can even license the technology so any fabricator can make it. We're going to be helping a lot of people!"

Which Dave is going to live a happier, more engaged, and productive life? The Dave who is bored and even embarrassed by his job, or the Dave who loves what he does and can't wait to talk about it?

IS IT YOUR JOB OR YOUR CAREER?

When you feel burned out, the very first question you should ask yourself is this:

"Am I burned out because of my *job* or my *career*?"

These are two very different things.

Your *job* is where you work *now*. It's your current employer.

Your *career* is your profession, what you do generally for a living.

For example, let's meet Susan. She's a medical billing and coding manager. That's her career. She earned a degree in accounting in college. She liked medical billing and coding, and she liked healthcare, so that's the industry in which she chose to work. She has dedicated herself to pursuing the highest professional standards in her field.

At the moment, Susan works for Sun Medical Billing and Coding. She's a senior manager overseeing a staff of 40 people. That's her job. When she graduated from college, she sent out a bunch of resumes, and Sun MB&C hired her. Hallelujah — she landed a good-paying job in the field she wanted to be in.

Susan has been with Sun MB&C for five years but the dream has turned sour. She's burned out. She hates coming to work in the morning. She feels alienated from her colleagues and disinterested in her department. Nothing of value seems to get done, at least in her view. Perhaps the workplace culture is even racist or sexist, or the company has been plagued by scandal or shoddy service.

At this point, Susan needs to think hard about what she wants. This should be her thought process:

Look Beyond Today's Paycheck

We all need money to live, but what we *think* we must bank every week can cloud our judgment. When you're feeling burned out and looking for a significant change, don't hesitate to look at the big picture and say, "Do I really need my level of income right now, or can I afford to take a chance?" This can be hard to do, especially if you're currently earning a comfortable salary and have the expenses, such as a mortgage, to match. But you must believe that if you're doing what you love in a positive environment, the money will take care of itself.

Consider Jeff Bezos, the founder of Amazon who is also no stranger to the title of wealthiest person on earth. You may not know the story of how he pursued and developed the idea for his online bookstore.

In his earlier life, Bezos had achieved spectacular success on Wall Street. A 1986 graduate of Princeton University with degrees in electrical engineering and computer science, Bezos was hired by Fitel, a telecommunications startup. From there, he went to Bankers Trust before landing a job at D.E. Shaw & Co., an emerging Wall Street hedge fund. He soon became a specialist in researching business opportunities in insurance, software, and the emerging internet. By the age of 30, Bezos had been promoted to senior vice president. At D.E. Shaw, he met fellow employee MacKenzie Scott, and they were married. By all accounts, Bezos and his wife were on the road to a very comfortable and lucrative career in finance.

In 1993, Bezos read a report that said the internet was growing at a rate of 2,300% a year. In addition, the U.S. government, which had exclusive control of the internet, was opening it up to private use. Sensing an opportunity, Bezos thought about building an online retail mail-order store. He didn't care much about what he sold; he chose books as the product because they were ubiquitous and easy to handle. The advantage of an internet store was that you could trim a few hours or days from the order-to-delivery timeline, and you didn't need an expensive bricks-and-mortar store. Your fulfillment center could be anywhere.

According to *Time* magazine, which named Bezos "Person of the Year" in 1999, Bezos pondered his decision in what he called his "regret-minimization framework." He imagined that he was 80 years old and looking back at his life. He realized his most important personal value wasn't just money; it was doing something meaningful. When he was 80, he imagined, he'd be okay with not receiving his six-figure Christmas bonus.

Most of all, he wouldn't regret having tried to build an online business and having failed. "In fact, I'd have been proud of that," he said. "Proud of myself for having taken that risk and tried to participate in that thing called the internet that I thought was going to be such a big deal. It was like the wild, wild West, a new frontier. And I knew that if I didn't try this, I would regret it. And that would be inescapable."

He calculated his odds of success at 30%. Luckily, his wife agreed to the crazy idea, and in 1994 the couple moved to a rented house in Seattle, Washington, and Bezos started looking for investors. He first approached his parents. As his stepfather Mike Bezos remembered, "When he called and said he wanted to sell books on the internet, we said, 'The internet? What's that?'" But they invested $300,000 to get him going and, in return, received 6% of a company that could have very quickly become worthless.[27]

The opposite happened. The Amazon website went live on July 16, 1995, and within two months, sales were up to $20,000 a week.

Make no mistake: Jeff Bezos was a smart guy, but he didn't know everything. He likes to tell a funny story about how he and his 10 employees, kneeling on the concrete floor of the garage, packed boxes of books for customers.

"I didn't have packing tables," he said at the Bush Center's Forum on Leadership in April 2018. "I said to one of the software engineers who was packing alongside me, 'You know what we should do? We should get knee pads.' And he looked at me like I was the dumbest guy he had ever seen in his life, and he said, 'Jeff, we should get packing tables.'"

Bezos later said getting packing tables was "the most brilliant idea" he had ever heard.

The next day, Bezos set up packing tables, and now the workers could stand up and move around easily. Bezos said the solution doubled their productivity.[28]

The rest, as they say, is history.

One thing to remember about Jeff Bezos is that when he was working on Wall Street, you couldn't say he was burned out and, therefore, needed a new direction. Bezos seems to be the kind of person who has the confidence to say, "What I'm doing now is acceptable, and I could probably keep doing it and be happy. But I want to have adventure in my life, and I don't want to settle for the ordinary because I'm too timid or risk-averse. If I fail, I can always get another job. But I have an opportunity, and I owe it to myself to take it." It's not always burnout that compels a person to make a change; sometimes, it's just seeing a door and saying to yourself, "I'm going to open that door and see what's on the other side."

If you're doing what you love, the expensive trappings of success will be much less important. Think about how many Hollywood stars achieve spectacular overnight success and immediately buy a huge $100 million mansion in the hills. For a few years, they try to manage their expensive castle, and then they quietly end up selling it for half of what they paid because they're glad to get rid of it. Many very successful people, like Warren Buffett, live in comfortable but not ostentatious houses because they don't want the headaches that come with a showplace.

It's sad when someone with training and education takes a job offer with a company they have misgivings about just because they think they must have a certain level of income. Such decisions rarely have good outcomes.

Ask Yourself What You Would Do if Every Job Paid the Same

Seriously, imagine that we lived in a weird sort of Utopia where every job paid the same. A janitor who worked eight hours a day received the same paycheck as the CEO. An inventor was paid the same as an orderly. A brain surgeon was paid the same as a nurse. The only variation was in your level of skill and experience; the more years you had on the job, the higher your paycheck. In this economy, the harder you worked, no matter your career, the more money you made.

If your current job were with the ideal company in your industry, would you keep it? For example, let's say Susan, the woman who manages a billing and coding office, is burned out and miserable at her job with Sun MB&C. Meanwhile, across town is Zenith Medical Billing, a company with a great reputation and a high score on Glassdoor. Susan's friend who works there tells her she should apply for an opening.

If Susan searched her soul and decided that she loved the medical billing and coding industry and everything about it, she would be wise to jump at the chance to change jobs and go to Zenith, even if it meant taking a cut in pay.

Identify the Source of Your Pain

"What is the source of my pain?" is your most important question. It may have more than one answer. In fact, make a list of the top things that bother you about your current work situation; the list can show anything, even things that you may think are trivial. Don't overanalyze it. Just grab a pen and paper and start writing.

Put at the top of the page: WHAT I HATE ABOUT MY JOB

Then, make your list. Let's say we asked Dave, the medical supply guy, to make his list. Perhaps this is what he would write:

1. The commute to work takes me over an hour. Too long.
2. My boss is no help. He just stays in his office all day. When we have a problem, he says we need to "figure it out."
3. Lousy benefits. The company pays only half of my health insurance, and I get only five sick days a year.
4. The boss hired his nephew, and the kid has zero qualifications. We have to cover for him.
5. Edna, the administrative assistant, cooks fish in the breakroom microwave. You can't go in there for an hour afterward.

If you look at Dave's list, you'll notice a few things.

Aside from his displeasure with the company benefits (#3), Dave does not complain about his paycheck. The omission indicates he believes he's being paid fairly for his work.

You'll also notice that he does not say anything negative about the work he does as a manufacturer of medical supplies. Every complaint — his commute, his boss, the benefits, the admin assistant — is about his *day-to-day job* at Acme Technology Corporation.

Dave gives no indication that he wants to leave the medical supplies industry. Dave's cure for his burnout might be to find a similar company to work for. This might be easy or it might be difficult. It needs to be closer to home, have better benefits, and offer a more supportive and positive company culture.

Dave knows what he wants; let's hope he can find it. If he lives in a rural area, there may not be another similar company within commuting distance, but if he lives in an area with lots of manufacturing, he might be able to make a change. Or he could move.

You could also look at the problem from the other side and ask Dave to list anything he *likes* about his current job.

WHAT I LOVE ABOUT MY JOB

1. We make very good products.
2. I like solving problems for our customers and making them happy.
3. I get to use my engineering skills.

Here, Dave reveals that he enjoys working within his industry. This confirms what we learned in the previous list: It's his current *job* he hates. Dave's next step is to research other job opportunities within his chosen career.

Let's say Sally, who also works at Acme Technology Corporation, feels burned out, just like Dave does. She makes a list of things she would change. This is her list:

WHAT I HATE ABOUT MY JOB

1. I have no interest in making exam gloves and feeding bags. Yuck!
2. I took this job because I needed a paycheck.
3. This place is noisy, and there are toxic chemicals in use.
4. Lifting heavy shipping boxes is bad for my back.
5. When can I retire and collect my Social Security?

You can see that, unlike Dave, Sally focuses all her complaints *on her career*. She never says anything bad about Acme Technology Corporation itself because the activities she dislikes are what she would experience at any similar company. Going to work for a different company in the same industry would make no difference; she'd still be miserable.

When asked to list the things she likes about her job, she says:

WHAT I LOVE ABOUT MY JOB

1. The people here are very nice.
2. The pay is good.
3. It's a short commute from my house.

We can see that the things she likes have nothing to do with her career, which confirms that getting a job with another company in the same industry would not make her happy.

Sally's next step is to research other careers she may want to enter. She may need to go back to school for training or start at an entry-level job and work her way up again.

We're not done yet; there's one more path that anyone could take. Let's look at a third person working at Acme Technology Corporation. Edward is also feeling burned out at his job. This is what his list looks like:

WHAT I HATE ABOUT MY JOB

1. Our newly released latex-free gloves are easily torn. We can do better.
2. Our supply chain is weak, and we often get defective parts from our suppliers.
3. We have too many products. We need to focus on what makes us a market leader.
4. Our website is confusing, and we lose sales when customers abandon their shopping carts.
5. Our industry relies too much on legacy technology. There's not enough innovation.

He also listed three things he loves about working at Acme Technology Corporation:

WHAT I LOVE ABOUT MY JOB

1. I enjoy managing the handful of entry-level employees who report to me.
2. My colleagues here are nice, but they need to be challenged.
3. The paycheck allows me to pay my bills.

We can see that Edward has a special view of his current job. To him, working at Acme Technology Corporation is not just a way to earn a paycheck or to use his degree in engineering; he's learning how to run a company, but he also sees the mistakes that are being made. Would Edward be happy finding a job at another company in the same industry? No, probably not. He's too ambitious. Does he want to leave his career and get a job in some other industry? No, there's no evidence of that. He has a keen interest in what he does for a living.

Edward's first step should be to try to work with his colleagues and managers to achieve change from within. Even if your company seems hopelessly difficult or out of touch, it's always possible that someone higher up feels the same way you do. In the 1990s, when General Motors exemplified the idea of a bastion of male superiority while its sales were tanking, is it possible that Mary Barra, who was then a manager of manufacturing planning in the Midsize Car Division, could have imagined herself as one day being the CEO and board chair? Probably not.

If that strategy fails, Edward might consider becoming an *entrepreneur*. That's a story we'll explore later in the book.

In our journey to find work/life synergy, where your work and your life are two sides of the same coin, we can safely say that if you're burned out at your job, then to support yourself and get happy again, you can choose from among three distinct paths:

1. Stay at your present job and find a way to make it work for you.
2. Change jobs by finding another role at a better company in the same industry.
3. Change your career by starting at an entry-level job, going back to school, or getting job training. You can also start your own business as an entrepreneur.

Let's look at each of the three paths.

CHAPTER 4

Path #1: Find Happiness in Your Present Job

THE FIRST PATH YOU CAN TAKE to survive burnout and achieve a satisfying work/life synergy is to stay in your present job and find a way to be happy.

To do this, you have two sources of power you can access: the power to effect change *within your company* and the power to effect change *within yourself.*

MAKE CHANGE WITHIN YOUR COMPANY

You may say to yourself, "The source of my burnout is my boss, or my colleagues, or the company culture. I want to keep working here, so I need to somehow get them to treat me fairly."

How can you make change within your company so that it's a better place to work?

Before you answer that, you must know what you expect and need from your workplace.

For example, for some people, being respected is their highest value. They don't care so much about being liked or having friends at work. Others put a premium on collegiality and feel as though their workplace is their second home. (We all know that person in the office who can be depended on to organize employee birthday parties.) Or they focus on achievement with a strong team and being able to go home at night with a feeling of accomplishment.

How people feel about the role of their workplace in their life colors how they perceive problematic decisions and attitudes. If all you want to do is keep your head down and take your paycheck, you may be very tolerant, but if you see yourself as a leader and a change agent, you'll be far more likely to try to change what you don't like or what seems unjust. Sometimes you may need to take strong steps and even file a lawsuit. Many corporate employees have sued their employer with the goal of changing the company culture; however, many who file suit do so *after* they've left the company. It's difficult to sue a company that you're still working for.

While a company's retaliation for complaints filed against it is a violation of federal law, details can get murky when your lawyer starts digging for the truth. Big companies have access to expensive lawyers, and cases can drag on for years, wearing down plaintiffs. For example, in 2018, 14 female former employees of Nike filed suit, describing the brand's headquarters in Beaverton, Oregon, as a "boys club" rife with sexual advances, suggestive comments, and other predatory behavior.

The lawsuit, which was unsealed in December 2022, included surveys by female employees of their peers in which the respondents described sexist attitudes and behavior at the sportswear giant, as well as fears of retaliation and corporate bullying. In one survey, obtained by *Business Insider*, an employee wrote that certain executives were "well-known philanderers with lower level employees whom they exert influence and power over," and one had been directed by male co-workers to "dress sexier." One female employee described Nike as "a giant men's sports team, where favoritism prevails, and females couldn't possibly play in the sandbox." Others said they doubted Nike's human-resources department would respond to their concerns.[29]

For its part, Nike says the company has improved pay equity and gender parity in executive positions. Soon after the scandal broke, Nike announced 7,000 workers would get raises. In 2022, women accounted for 43% of vice-presidents at the company, up from 36% in 2018. Nike is a big company, and it's difficult to gauge how much a lawsuit like this brought in measurable change, but one thing you know is true: The women who filed the lawsuit are feeling very good about themselves because they took action to change the culture of their company.

The confrontational path can be difficult, especially if you hope to remain employed at the same company. It's challenging for an employee to leverage change from within because the people responsible for the culture are the leaders and owners, and if they want to get rid of you, they can find a way.

Recently, there's been a lot of talk about *managing up,* a strategy whereby an employee can reduce the negative effects of a manager who has human shortcomings. In a sense, it's a way to avoid burnout by keeping one step ahead of it. You make a little extra effort *now* to avoid a bigger effort or emotional stress *later.*

The strategy involves anticipating what the boss wants and then giving it to them. For example, if the boss wants a one-page summary report every morning, you make sure he gets it, even if you think it's unnecessary. He'll be happy and won't pester you for the report. If your boss is forgetful, send little reminders. If she's having a bad day, offer to stay late and help her. All of these measures are things you can do to make your life easier in the future.

Harvard Business Review puts it this way: "Bad bosses are the stuff of legend. And too many managers are overextended, overwhelmed, or downright incompetent — a topic that HBR has covered extensively over the years. Even if your boss has some serious shortcomings, it's in your best interest, and it's your responsibility, to make the relationship work."[30]

One respected expert says, "If you notice your manager dealing with extra stress and pressure, offer to help them run a team meeting or take on an additional task to reduce their workload."[31]

This can be an effective way to create a smoothly running workplace and reduce burnout, but it should be approached with common sense. You cannot hope to fix a serious problem with company management over which you have no control. Think about especially egregious cases, like the infamous case when Wells Fargo forced its employees to commit fraud in order to meet impossible sales goals. How exactly could those employees have improved their situation by managing up? The rot extended right up to the office of CEO John Stumpf. If employees didn't go along with the illicit scheme, they were fired.

This book is not about allowing yourself to be a victim. It's about conducting yourself with dignity and having respect for others, loving what you do every day to support yourself, and ending each day with a happy heart. At some point, it may mean saying, "I'm not going to invest my time and energy in a bad situation. I need to get out."

Only you can know when to say, "I'm going to get out." Change does not happen overnight, and there are many cases in which people decide to have faith in the future, stay with their employer, rise up through the ranks, and then use their authority to make improvements for everyone.

Let's imagine that Dave, our medical devices company friend, decides to stay with Acme Technology Corporation because he simply cannot find another job in his career field. In the medical equipment business, Acme is the "only game in town," and Dave doesn't want to uproot his family by moving. He makes the decision to somehow be happy at Acme, climb the corporate ladder, become CEO, and remake the company into what he thinks it ought to be.

In this regard, his career path would be similar to that of Mary Barra at General Motors. She began working at GM at the age of 18 as a hood and fender inspector. She worked her way up through the ranks until January 15, 2014, when, at the age of 53, she was named the first female CEO of a major auto manufacturer. She doesn't talk about it, but you can only imagine what she must have gone through as she rose higher in the male-dominated world of auto manufacturing, especially through the dismal period of bankruptcy when it seemed as though the company might collapse.

Upon taking the helm of the revived automaker, she set about changing the company culture. One of her first edicts as CEO was to eliminate the highly detailed GM dress code and replace it with two words: "Dress appropriately." She also issued a succinct directive for her 216,000 company employees: "No more crappy cars."

She has said a few things about avoiding burnout. As she explained at an event hosted by *The Wall Street Journal*, she does not book meetings at dinnertime. Instead, she'll schedule work lunches, which she says allows her (and others) to have better work/life synergy. Barra also prioritizes her family obligations in the same way she does her work commitments. She explained, "I'll say, 'The meeting starts at 4:30, and it's going to end at 5:30 because I'm making my child's sporting event.' Everyone says, 'OK, let's be efficient, let's get this done.'"[32]

Ask yourself: To what extent are your feelings of being burned out caused by specific conditions at your workplace? If they are, do you have any power to change them? Can you ask your manager for help? Do you think your company leaders have the awareness and empathy they need to make the workplace healthier?

WORKING HAPPY THROUGH ADVERSITY

We all face challenges in our workplace or career path, especially if we're entering a field that's well-entrenched and may be difficult for newcomers to enter and thrive. If you happen to be in a situation where you're facing outright opposition to your presence, but you love your work and are determined to succeed, you'll need a thick skin. You'll need to be like a cheerful little armadillo, protected by her tough hide, marching forward, never giving up, always seeing the good and ignoring the bad.

Consider Katherine Johnson, who was the subject of the popular film *Hidden Figures*. Born on August 26, 1918, as a child, she showed evidence of being a prodigy in math, and her parents, although they were not wealthy, ensured that she received a good education. At the age of 14, she graduated from high school and enrolled in West Virginia State College, an historically black college. Regarding discrimination, she said, "I didn't have time for that. My dad taught us, 'You are as good as anybody in this town, but you're no better.' I don't have a feeling of inferiority. Never had. I'm as good as anybody, but no better."[33]

In 1937, at age 18, Johnson graduated *summa cum laude* with degrees in mathematics and French. This was at a time when just 2% of black women got a university degree, and more than half of those became teachers. Johnson took on a teaching job at a black public school in Marion, Virginia, but she wanted to become a research mathematician, a career field rife with discrimination against women and blacks.

Her career took off in 1953 when the National Advisory Committee for Aeronautics (NACA) hired her to be one of several women in the Guidance and Navigation Department. The women were called "computers," which is funny because, in those days, there were no computers as we know them, just people with slide rules. (If you're too young to know what a slide rule is, just Google it.) Like that of the other women, Johnson's job was to make fast and accurate mathematical calculations relating to aeronautics. This was regarded as "women's work," while the men handled the actual engineering questions.

By 1946, the Langley Research Center had recruited about 400 female human computers. Johnson's workplace at Langley was subject to Virginia's Jim Crow laws and racially segregated; Johnson and the other black female computers worked in the all-black West Area Computing section, while the white computers worked in the East section.

Johnson found ways to assert her humanity. She refused to obey the segregated bathroom rules and avoided eating in the segregated cafeteria. During breaks, she talked about aviation magazines and played cards with her white male colleagues. She even successfully demanded that she be allowed to attend high-level briefings — and her white male colleagues were compelled to accede because the quality of her work made her presence not only tolerable but necessary.

In 1958, NACA became part of the National Aeronautics and Space Administration (NASA), which was officially desegregated, and Johnson became a key numbers cruncher; however, discrimination continued, and during her early years at NASA, Johnson could not even put her name on any reports — her own work product — because she was a woman. Eventually, her male boss was forced to put her name on a report about orbital flight because her contribution was important and undeniable.

Among other historical tasks, using her trusty slide rule and adding machine, she did trajectory analysis for America's first human spaceflight, Alan Shepard's Freedom 7 mission in May 1961. At a time when digital computers were relatively new and untested, she checked the computer's math for John Glenn's historic first orbital spaceflight by an American in February 1962. Glenn had personally insisted that Johnson review the electronic computer's calculations as a prerequisite to his agreeing to be hurtled into space. In 1969, she performed the calculations for the first moon landing.

Johnson worked on the space shuttle program until 1986, then spent her retirement encouraging students to enter the fields of science, technology, engineering, and mathematics. She died in 2020 at the age of 101. The mother of three daughters, Johnson is a shining example of someone who enjoyed an almost perfect work/life synergy. She entered a profession that was openly racist and sexist, but she stayed laser-focused on her special gift and was so good at what she did that she *forced the organization to adapt to her.*

This does not mean that a black woman, or any minority person for that matter, needs to be superhuman to earn fair treatment. That would be absurd. Fair treatment must be available to everybody, but we can thank Katherine Johnson and the other black women "computers" for being strong enough to break down walls purely by the force of their will.

MAKE CHANGE WITHIN YOURSELF

The other way to survive burnout at your current job is to change yourself from within. Once again, it does *not* mean accepting an abusive job situation. It does *not* mean becoming a victim. It means finding as much good as you can in your job and career and having a personal goal that keeps you motivated during difficult times.

How can you do this? There are several strategies you can use. As you'll see in this chapter, we discuss how to avoid burnout if you're an employee at a mid- or large-sized organization with many workers. In such an environment, it's your job to get along with those who have authority over you, including the board of directors and your colleagues, with whom you must have a smooth and frictionless working relationship.

In the previous section, we discussed how you can try to change your organization from within. In this section, we'll examine how you can thrive by changing yourself from within, embracing the best parts of your role, setting limits, and staying healthy.

Become an "Organization Person"

To thrive and achieve work/life synergy, you first need to know yourself. This may seem like a question that's almost too simple, but have you ever thought deeply about whether you see yourself as a self-employed entrepreneur or as a person who works better in a large group? This is a valid question for nearly any industry. You can be a doctor and have your own practice, which brings its own burnout challenges, or you can work for a big hospital, which brings different burnout challenges. You could be a lawyer in private practice or practice with a big firm. You could be a writer and be self-employed or work for a national media company.

All these situations have the potential for burnout, but in different ways. If you work for an organization, the source of your burnout is likely to be your boss and, to some extent, your co-workers. If you're self-employed, you're your own boss, and if you're burned out, you need only look in the mirror to see who's responsible!

A key question you need to ask yourself is, "Do I feel happier and more productive in a group or on my own?"

In 1956, author William H. Whyte explored this question in his book *The Organization Man*, which became a bestseller and one of the most influential books ever written on management.

The book came about when Whyte, while employed by *Fortune* magazine, did a series of interviews with CEOs of major American corporations such as General Electric and Ford. A central theme of the book was that average Americans were shifting from the prevailing notion of rugged individualism to a collectivist ethic, that people believed that organizations and groups could make better decisions than individuals, and thus, serving an organization was a better choice than trying to forge an individual path.

Whyte believed this to be incorrect and described how individual work and creativity had produced better outcomes than collectivist processes. This was the age of middle management when conformity was prized, and the standard uniform of the businessman (women were not part of the equation) was the blue or grey suit, white button-down shirt, and necktie.

You may or may not agree with Whyte's viewpoint, but his portrait of the Organization Man was interesting. Today, we talk about the Organization Person as someone who thrives within an organization and enjoys the collaboration and team focus that are hallmarks of an effective organization of any type. The Organization Person also enjoys, or at least tolerates, the tribal backstabbing and double-dealing that are a part of most profit-driven organizations. The successful Organization Person is also keenly aware of the most prominent liability of organizations: lack of innovation, embrace of the *status quo*, and criticism of those who are perceived as non-conformists.

Let's return to our friend Mary Barra, who is clearly the quintessential Organization Person. She has obviously thrived within the vast beehive of General Motors, whose very name suggests bland conformity, and has found a way to exert her vision for the company across its 167,000 employees. In all of her interviews, she has never once suggested that she disliked working at GM or had considered employment elsewhere.

It helps that she's a "car gal." She loves cars, always has, and harbors a deep personal interest in the products made by her company. Her husband drives a Chevy Camaro, their son has a Pontiac Firebird, and the family owns a Hummer. As of 2022, Barra herself was driving a Chevy Bolt EV, which anyone could buy for less than $30,000.

You never know who might thrive within an organization. For example, Steve Jobs co-founded Apple and helped build it into a significant company until 1985, when an internal power struggle with then-CEO John Sculley led to his ouster. At that point, it would have been easy to conclude that the volatile, eccentric Jobs was *not* an Organization Person and could not function within a company that at that time had 5,000 employees.

In 1997, Jobs returned to Apple as CEO. The company now had 8,400 employees but was on the verge of bankruptcy. He is credited with reviving Apple, and by the time he left for health reasons in 2011, the company had grown to over 60,000 employees and had a market capitalization of $297 billion. Clearly, to accomplish what he did, this unpredictable and demanding innovator had significant strengths as an Organization Person.

He was succeeded by Tim Cook, who in many ways was seen as the opposite of Jobs: introverted, low-key, almost mousy. Most analysts predicted that without the fiery presence of Steve Jobs, the company had seen its best days. Tim Cook, they said, was too weak to take charge of such a cutting-edge technology firm.

Tim Cook proved them wrong and thrived as Apple's CEO. By 2021, 10 years after the death of Steve Jobs, Apple had grown to 164,000 employees, with a market cap of nearly $3 trillion and $62 billion in free cash — the most of any company.[34]

If you're burned out at work, it may mean that you don't *see yourself* as an Organization Person, at least not with your current employer. But perhaps you could become one. If you do, the most important things to remember are the three rules, which apply to any job, but especially to a job to which you may not be totally in love:

1. Resist efforts by management to work you like a farm animal. Some companies have no regard for the welfare of their employees. Don't feel guilty about asserting your rights.

2. Focus on what you're doing that pleases you, such as making customers happy. The thing about customers is that they don't care about the behind-the-scenes drama at your workplace. They pay their money, and they expect good service and quality products. Remember them as you work.

3. Fly above internal politics. Make no alliances and make no enemies. Commit to doing the job you're hired to do and give no support to people who are negative or divisive. If you are the target of racist or sexist attacks, only you can decide if you can — or should — ignore them and keep marching forward. You can train yourself to become emotionally detached from practices that have offended you in the past and take an attitude of "I'm just going to float over it, keep a smile on my face, and get on with my life."

In such a case, *succeeding within the challenging environment at work* becomes one of the missions of your life. It's what will give you personal satisfaction in much the same way as shooting under par on the golf course or completing a marathon. Everyone has personal goals, whether it's ensuring a child goes to college, paying off the home mortgage, or bowling a perfect 300 game. Setting goals helps you develop new behaviors, sharpen your focus, and increase your momentum in life. Your goals should be value-based, meaning they're tied to the overall health and well-being of you, your family, and your community. Goals that are shallow, such as "make more money," are more difficult to sustain.

Your personal goal could be to navigate your way through the challenging job environment and come out on top. For some people, playing the game of corporate chutes and ladders is enjoyable.

Ask yourself: Do you enjoy working with a team where there's a hierarchy? This is a situation in which you have a boss who can direct your work, colleagues with whom you must cooperate, and perhaps subordinates who report to you. If you enjoy that, or if you have no choice because of your job options, then you can develop skills that will help you succeed. You can focus on the good parts, rise above the bad parts, and look at your situation with an objective eye.

CHAPTER 5

Path #2: Change Jobs

THIS IS PRETTY STRAIGHTFORWARD. You like the work that you do, just not the company, so you take your existing skills and experience and move them to an environment that you hope will be more conducive to your work/life synergy. Your career remains the same; it's where you earn your paycheck that changes.

You would do this because, for one or more reasons, you believe you cannot fix or make your present situation better. Reasons include:

No path upward. Here, while you may enjoy your work and have no problem with the company itself, you're looking to the future. You're probably at a small company with fewer than a hundred employees, and it may be family-owned or headed by the founder. Looking around you, it's clear that either other people have been anointed as successors to the current leadership or the leaders are likely to sell the business when they retire.

In any case, your opportunities for career and income growth are slight. You can choose to stay with the company until you retire, which, if you're happy, might be the best choice for you, or you can bail out and jump to another firm with better prospects for career growth.

In this scenario, you may not even be burned out. You're just making a change to *avoid* becoming burned out in the future. You're being smart; you can make the move while you have time to make the right choice. Take your time, continue to provide excellent service to your current employer, don't burn any bridges, and leave on good terms.

Long commute. Commuting to work can be:
1. Incredibly boring because you must creep along a highway jammed with cars. You could almost get there faster if you walked!

2. Incredibly stressful because you're forced to hurtle down the highway while pursued by crazy drivers who seem determined to win the race to get to work.

3. Both boring and stressful, depending upon the day and time.

For millions of workers, commuting is no fun, and changing jobs because of a long commute is increasingly common. In 2018, before the COVID-19 pandemic, global staffing firm Robert Half surveyed more than 2,800 Americans across 28 major U.S. cities and found that 23% of workers, surprisingly men more likely than women, had quit a job because of a bad commute.[35]

The drive is getting longer. According to the U.S. Census Bureau, the average commute time in 1990 was less than 22 minutes each way. By 2021, Americans were spending 25.6 minutes of commute time to work each way. These extra 3.6 minutes of commute time may seem trivial, but they add up to roughly 30 more hours per year sitting in your car or on the train.[36]

What could you do with 30 extra hours? You could watch 15 feature films, attend 10 NFL football games, read three classic novels, or even sit through one major league baseball game (just kidding!).

While the office's overachiever who walks or bikes to work minds it the least, for most of us, time spent driving to work or riding the train is time wasted. A study by the University of the West of England, which analyzed the impact of commuting on more than 26,000 employees in England over a five-year period, found that each extra minute of commuting by car or train reduced the job and leisure time satisfaction of workers, increased their strain, and worsened their mental health.

The chief culprits for long commutes were boredom and being sedentary. "We know that regularly driving for more than two to three hours a day is bad for your heart," commented Kishan Bakrania, an epidemiologist who worked on the report. "This research suggests it is bad for your brain, too, perhaps because your mind is less active in those hours."[37]

A long commute can be a major contributor to workplace burnout — and a drag on your health. Studies have shown that people with commutes of 20 miles or more have greater rates of high blood pressure and high blood sugar than those with short commutes. While these negative effects may seem to be nothing more than the cost of our modern life, after sitting in traffic for long stretches of time, many people lose their willpower to exercise. One study found that people who spent more time commuting consistently spent less time exercising, sleeping, and making food at home. They were also more likely to buy "non-grocery food purchases" (that is, fast food or takeout).[38] Not good for the health!

To shorten your commuting time while staying at your present job, you might ask your boss whether any part of your job can be done remotely. Shortening the workweek, even periodically, can reduce your weekly commute time and, as a bonus, shrink your global carbon footprint. According to a U.K. study conducted by Platform London, implementing a four-day workweek by 2025 would reduce Britain's carbon emissions by more than 20%. It would reduce energy use in the workplace and slash vehicle emissions by cutting back on commuting. It also found that giving people an extra day off increased the amount of "low-carbon" activities they enjoy, including resting, exercising, community-building, and seeing family, thus reducing overall consumption.[39]

It's a personal decision, but if by working at or near your home helps you achieve work/life synergy, you may not only be happier but also healthier.

Intolerable culture. People often change jobs because, despite their best efforts, they simply cannot tolerate how they're treated at work. For them, working happy with good work/life synergy is not possible at their present place of employment.

You've heard the saying, "Employees don't quit their jobs; they quit their managers." Of course, while not an exact science, there's evidence to suggest this is a credible adage.

In 2021, Gallup published its *State of the American Workplace* report based on data collected from more than 195,600 U.S. employees, more than 31 million respondents, and insight from leading

Fortune 1000 companies. In the report, Gallup CEO Jim Clifton underscored the importance of managers in creating a positive company culture that promotes employee retention. Speaking to CEOs, he wrote, "The single biggest decision you make in your job — bigger than all the rest — is whom you name manager. When you name the wrong person manager, nothing fixes that bad decision. Not compensation, not benefits — nothing."[40]

Among the many relationships you'll develop at a company, those formed with your manager have a significant impact on your overall workplace experience, even more so than your relationships with your peers.

But the fact is that while most leaders want their team members to learn and thrive, others may feel threatened by those they believe are too competent and could probably do their job better than them. Research shows that in such cases, managers can react aggressively and say or do things that make their jealousy evident. Such a manager might:

- Belittle your accomplishments in front of your team.
- Enjoy pointing out your mistakes.
- Interrupt you during meetings or one-on-ones.
- Ignore you.
- Frequently find something to criticize about your work.
- Assign you projects no one else wants to work on.[41]

If this is your situation, your manager may have identified you as a threat to them. If you cannot "manage up" and reduce the tension, your only choice might be to leave.

You cannot use your best skills. This is very common. The job isn't challenging, and you're simply bored. This may not be the fault of the company; you may have reached the limit of what the company can offer, and the leadership is happy with the *status quo*. However, you feel the burnout creeping up on you, and you decide you need a change.

According to the Gallup report, 60% of employees say the ability to do what they do best in a role is "very important" to them. Workers want employers who allow them to make the most of their strengths in their roles. They do their best in roles that enable them to integrate their knowledge (what they know), skills (what they can do), and talent (the natural capacity for excellence).

It's a two-way street; "what I do best" means matching the role and culture with the right person. When an employee is a mismatch for their role and organization, they often become bored and restless, or the opposite: they struggle to succeed. Their workdays, even their entire careers, can feel wasted, with no emotional reward or sense of purpose.[42]

If you find yourself "quietly quitting" or feeling like your current job is unfulfilling or a dead end, you owe it to yourself to seek greener pastures elsewhere.

FINDING A COMPANY YOU LIKE

Should you decide to make a change, your challenge is to find an organization where you'll be a good fit, and you'll be working happy. If you're not careful, you may jump from the frying pan into the fire and find yourself in a situation just as unpleasant, if not worse, than the one you left behind.

Unless your reason for switching companies is a straightforward one like a shorter commute or because your manager has switched companies and wants you to follow her, you need to proceed with caution and try to find out as much as you can about the firm you're interested in.

The plain fact is this: Just as job applicants put their best foot forward when selling themselves to their prospective employers, hiring managers do the same thing. They're not going to tell you the company has a horrendous employee turnover rate or is fighting multiple race discrimination cases, or the previous CEO was quietly given a golden parachute and shown the door because of some sort of misconduct.

Such firings happen, as in 2019, when fast-food giant McDonald's dismissed CEO Steve Easterbrook for violating company policy by having a consensual relationship with an employee. But he was not fired "for cause," which meant he was still able to walk away with a severance package estimated to be $105 million.

How can you peer behind the culture curtain of the company you might be joining and have some assurance you won't get burned out in a year or two?

You need to put on your investigative hat and do some research.

Google Them!

The first thing to do is the most obvious: Google the company. (Or Bing, Baidu, or Yahoo! — your choice.) See what you find in the "news" category.

For example, in February 2023, I Googled "Twitter" because the company had been in the news for the past few months. Hypothetically, if someone had offered me a job there — which was not going to happen — what I saw would not have been encouraging. The headlines blared:

"In Latest Round of Job Cuts, Twitter Is Said to Lay Off at Least 200 Employees." – *The New York Times.*

"Elon Musk lays off more Twitter employees, including hardcore loyalists: 'Looks like I'm let go.'" – *Yahoo Finance.*

"Esther Crawford, Twitter exec who slept in office overnight, is fired: report." – *The New York Post.*

"Twitter Glitches Pile Up as Key Features Fail." – *The New York Times.*

In terms of the employment outlook and company culture, nothing in the news was encouraging. In all fairness, companies can change, and if you're really interested in working there, you have little to lose by interviewing and seeing what they tell you.

Big companies like Twitter, now X, are newsworthy and covered by the press, but your Google search for a small company may not bring up anything other than the firm's website and a few routine press releases. Either way, you have additional investigative tools at your disposal.

Glassdoor

The next place you can look is Glassdoor. This website is the leading "town square" where real employees of real companies provide insight into what it's like to actually work there. The service it provides is worthwhile because the gap between what the company wants you to believe and what employees experience can be wide.

A survey by Glassdoor revealed that 61% of respondents found aspects of a new job different than what they had expected based on the interview process. Company culture, employee morale, job responsibilities, and boss's personality were cited as some of the factors that differed most between the interview and the actual work site.[43]

Of course, you can't believe everything you read on the internet, including anonymous postings, but you can get a feeling and a "vibe" from big sites like Glassdoor. The site also ranks companies based on employee reviews; the company claims, "Winners are determined solely based on feedback provided by those who really know a company best — the employees. There is no nomination process, no employee surveys or questionnaires and no costs or fees involved."

The website lists over 450,000 companies, including more than 380,000 that have been rated in the category of work/life balance.[44]

Indeed

Indeed.com has over 300 million unique visitors every month. The site provides free access to job searches, posted resumes, and research companies. Uniquely, it provides the "Work Happiness Score" based on 15 dimensions of work happiness, which helps you "find a place where you belong."

Just for fun, I searched for ABC Supply Co. Inc., headquartered just down the street from where I work in Beloit, Wisconsin. It's the largest wholesale distributor of roofing in the United States and the nation's largest distributor of select exterior and interior building products, tools, and related supplies. With over 860 locations in 49 states supported by more than 17,000 employees, ABC Supply has a reputation as one of the most desirable workplaces in the world.

I was delighted to learn that as a 14-time winner of the Gallup Great Workplace Award, it's one of only three companies across the globe to receive the honor each year since its inception in 2007. ABC Supply is also a Glassdoor Employees' Choice Award winner.

While I was aware of the company, little did I know that it was so highly regarded!

CHAPTER 6

Path #3: Change Your Career

WILL YOU STAY IN THE SAME INDUSTRY for your entire career, or at some point, will you make a big shift?

Only you can answer that question.

Before we dive into the question of a career change, we should first recognize that there are no clear statistics regarding how often people change careers as opposed to just changing jobs.

I define *a career as* continuous work in a defined industry, such as healthcare. A *job* is a defined role in a particular company. At a hospital, non-clinical jobs would include receptionists, medical billers and coders, hospital executives, transcriptionists, as well as anyone who works behind the scenes, such as IT, administrative assistants, human resources personnel, biomedical technicians, and more.

You can change jobs within one company or between companies in the same industry. But if you change industries, that's a career change.

One more note: The healthcare industry, about which this book is the focus, is so broad and diffuse that the thousands of non-clinical healthcare jobs overlap with many other industries. Administrators, billers, IT people, and insurance experts have fungible skills that are easily transferable to other industries. If you work in human resources at a big hospital, you could easily make the jump to just about any other large company. The basic employment laws and practices are the same. But if you're in a clinical position, it can be different. If you're a brain surgeon, the places you can work are limited. If you're an orthopedist, on the other hand, you could move out of a hospital setting and get a job with a college or professional sports team. So the lines between careers and industries can be fuzzy.

Given that uncertainty, we'll forge ahead.

While the U.S. Bureau of Labor Statistics tracks the number of *job* changes of the average American, it does not track a person's *career* changes in a lifetime. This is because it's difficult to define what a career change is. Is going from working as the endowment manager in a nonprofit hospital to becoming a trader on Wall Street a career change? No one is sure. However, for practical purposes, experts say the average number of lifetime career changes is four, while the average number of job changes an American employee makes is 12. This suggests that every third job an employee takes is also a career change.

Some people embark on their career path early in life, sometimes even in high school, and settle into a work/life synergy that remains the same for decades or even an entire lifetime. For some reason, these "early careerists" find their passion in life quickly and pursue it without getting bored, burned out, or feeling they've done all they can and are in need of a change.

History provides us with examples of such people, many of whom are artists. Pablo Picasso, for instance, showed exceptional ability in drawing and painting by the age of seven. He attended art school, and for the duration of his 91 years, he was never anything but a self-employed artist.

Bill Gates is an example of an early careerist from the technology sector. At age 13, he wrote his first software program. At 17, Gates, with his friend Paul Allen, formed a partnership called Traf-O-Data, which supplied traffic data to generate reports for traffic engineers. In the autumn of 1973, he entered Harvard University. Two years later, he dropped out to form Microsoft, where he served for 35 years as CEO; in 2008, he transitioned to a part-time role. In 2014, Gates stepped down as chairman of the board, and in 2020, he left the board entirely, ending his 45-year association with the company he founded.

Not all early careerists are famous. A recent internet search brought up stories about many people who were retiring after 50 years or more in the same career. For example, in 2022, TMJ4 News in Milwaukee reported on a man named Tom Bonesho, who retired after working for half a century in local grocery stores. He got his first job at the age of 16, bagging groceries. He spent the rest of his career in a wide variety of supermarket roles in his community. "I've done everything," he said. "I've done pricing, I've run the office, I ran the bakery, the deli departments. I was a dairy manager, frozen foods. Yeah, I know the business, I think."[45]

I don't know Tom personally, but he sounds like a person who achieved lasting work/life synergy. The key may have been the fact that while he loved the grocery industry, he held a wide variety of jobs within it. He never got bored because he regularly changed jobs and acquired new skills.

Some early careerists who achieve a highly productive work/life synergy don't *change* careers so much as *add* to them. Richard Branson is someone who keeps adding more activities to his business portfolio. At age 20, he began his first successful venture with a mail-order record business, which soon became Virgin Records. Always a restless entrepreneur, over the years, he expanded the Virgin brand to include Virgin Atlantic airline, the Virgin Rail Group, Virgin Hotels, and many more. In 2004, he founded space-flight corporation Virgin Galactic. As of 2023, his Virgin Group included more than 40 companies across five business sectors and five continents. (Alas, Virgin Records was not one of them; in 1992, he sold it to EMI.)

In his case, as with many other serial entrepreneurs, it's safe to say that Branson would describe his life mission as starting new businesses. Unlike many other entrepreneurs, while Branson has sold (or "exited") some of his businesses, his tendency is to turn them over to managers while retaining an ownership stake. By doing that, he can remain involved in a directorial role.

While some people are early careerists, many follow a more meandering trajectory. There are no rules for how a human life should unfold, and many people change careers several times in their lives. They do this for any one of four reasons.

THE FOUR REASONS PEOPLE CHANGE CAREERS

1. They're Burned Out

These people work for a substantial length of time in their chosen career and, for various reasons, become unhappy with their current state and need a new purpose to their life. A career that once was in alignment with their purpose is no longer fulfilling, and therefore, the sacrifices they made for that career, such as working long hours, seem pointless. Even a high salary is not enough to make them happy.

When your heart isn't in your work, it becomes drudgery. We'll talk much more about your purpose or your "why" in the pages ahead.

2. They've Gone as Far as Their Current Career Can Take Them

No matter how enjoyable they may be, many careers are limited in what you elicit from them personally, such as how much money you can make or the skills you can acquire. When some people reach the top level of their career path, rather than remaining in place, they switch to a new path that will lead them to a higher place of personal achievement.

Arnold Schwarzenegger is one of those people. He emigrated from his native Austria to the United States at the age of 21, having already won the title of Mr. Universe as a bodybuilder. His ambition was to become the greatest bodybuilder in the world, and two years later, he became the youngest man to win the Mr. Olympia competition. (It seems that in the world of bodybuilding, Olympia is bigger than Universe.)

But no matter how successful you are, a career as a bodybuilder has its limits, so Schwarzenegger set his sights on becoming a movie star — not because he was burned out with bodybuilding but because he had reached the top and had nowhere to go. Against the odds of his unusual name and thick Austrian accent being seen as career-killers, he was cast in films and starred in a string of blockbusters that made him a global superstar. In 1993, the National Association of Theatre Owners named him the "International Star of the Decade."

That was his second act, and for most people, it would have been enough, but Schwarzenegger set his sights on an even bigger third act. In 1990, he became involved in Republican Party politics, and in 2003 was elected governor of California. In 2006, he won re-election and served until 2011. Many people believe that if Schwarzenegger had been a native-born American, he would have run for President, but alas, he's ineligible.

Schwarzenegger might have been someone who said, "This is who I am, and I need the world to realize that and make a place for me." But he was *realistic* in that he knew the world did not owe him a living and *opportunistic* in his eagerness to try new things. In fact, when he first arrived in America, he had to make money, so in 1968, he and fellow bodybuilder Franco Columbu started a bricklaying business.

The business flourished, and they rolled over the profits to start a mail-order business selling bodybuilding and fitness-related equipment and instructional tapes. He plowed the profits from the mail-order business and his bodybuilding competition winnings into his first real estate investment, an apartment building he purchased for $10,000; further investment in a number of real estate holding companies resulted in his currently significant real estate portfolio.

Schwarzenegger exemplifies someone who knew how to work happy and avoid burnout for two reasons: (1) He never lost sight of why he was working, and (2) He was happy to change his goal when the time was right.

If you can do that, you're virtually guaranteed to be working happy!

3. They "Age Out" of a Successful Career

Some careers are "evergreen," meaning you can follow them at any age. Author Stephen King, who, as of this writing, is 75 years old, has been happily doing the same work for over 50 years. Workers in our industrial society can hold onto most jobs until retirement and even longer, but a few jobs come with a soft age limit, particularly those of professional athletes who cross an age threshold after which they can no longer safely or profitably compete. (This would have happened to Schwarzenegger, but he got out of bodybuilding competitions before he would have started losing them.)

Most athletes can play only until their 30s. Tom Brady, hailed as the greatest football quarterback of all time, lasted until his retirement at age 45. In May 2022, a year before his final season, Brady signaled his career change by signing an unprecedented 10-year, $375 million deal to become a football TV analyst for the Fox Television network, which airs NFL games. This will be his second act, but at the end of his decade-long deal in 2033, he'll be only 56 years old — and ready for act three.

4. They Need New Challenges

For some people, satisfaction comes from the journey, not the destination. They launch a business, bring it to a certain level, then exit and start another business. There are many such serial entrepreneurs, and it might be argued that they don't really change careers because their chosen career path is to start new businesses. That's their purpose.

Richard Branson is one of those restless entrepreneurs who seeks new challenges as an antidote to becoming burned out. Another entrepreneur is Oprah Winfrey, who was fired as a newscaster for becoming too emotionally involved with the stories, launched her own TV afternoon talk show, and went on to found Harpo Productions, then television cable station Oxygen Media and several other print and publishing companies, including O, The Oprah Magazine. She also owns OWN, the Oprah Winfrey Channel, where she produces and stars in various TV shows and movies.

And there is Jeff Bezos, who by all accounts was perfectly happy with his high-paying job on Wall Street, but when he learned of the enormous potential of the internet, he knew he had to take a chance and embark on a new career. Once Amazon became profitable, he expanded the business to Amazon Web Services (cloud computing), Zoox (autonomous vehicles), Kuiper Systems (satellite internet), and Amazon Lab126 (computer hardware R&D). Other subsidiaries include Ring, Twitch, IMDb, and Whole Foods Market. In addition, Bezos is the founder of aerospace company Blue Origin and owner of The Washington Post newspaper.

Many people noted here have become extremely wealthy as a result of their career aspirations. That's not going to happen to everyone, because most people don't have that rare combination of specialized skills, ambition, and opportunity. But anyone can feel the irrepressible urge to seek a better life. If you're experiencing job burnout and you believe that changing companies within the same industry would not make you happy, one solution is to stay in your current career and add a side venture.

ADD A SIDE VENTURE OR PRODUCTIVE HOBBY

Many people who face burnout adopt a hybrid solution: They stick with their current job and career path, but they start another venture into which they can pour their imagination and extra energy, or they get a part-time job in another industry, or they develop a productive hobby (that is to say, something more substantial than playing golf). For example, many working people get involved in real estate, either as agents or as investors. They can pursue this in their free time during the evening and on weekends. They can build it over time and perhaps even someday make it their main job.

This strategy provides three benefits:

1. It separates your current job from the rest of your life and makes it easier to walk away from it at the end of the workday. Let's explain what that means. Because the goal of this book is to help you achieve a happy work/life synergy, you might assume that a primary condition is that you love every aspect of your 9 to 5 job. Actually, that may never happen. No job is perfect, and even the best jobs can be boring or difficult once in a while.

   No matter what your job is, it's important that you're able to leave it behind when the sun sets. This helps you to go in fresh the next morning, But if you have no other responsibilities after work, you're likely to allow yourself to acquiesce to after-work demands. This leads to burnout.

   On the other hand, if you're deeply involved in something else, such as a part-time job, a hobby, or a new venture, then it's easier to turn off your mind from your regular job. In other words, a side gig can enhance your tolerance for your regular job because it's no longer the absolute center of your life. You may be tired from working long hours, but you'll be happier than if you had gone home and watched TV.

71

2. While a hobby will probably cost you money, a side gig can provide income. This will ease some pressure and help you to work happy. It may also grow to become a sufficient amount to allow you to go into it full-time.

   Unfortunately, many people need to work multiple jobs just to pay the bills; they have no choice. This is a difficult situation to be in, and in terms of working happy, the best you can do is try to find work that provides you with satisfaction but keep your eye on the big picture, which is the fact that you're providing a better future for your family.

3. If your regular job provides sufficient stable income — if not a satisfactory work/life synergy — then you can explore your new interest without the worry of having to make it support you. People who don't need extra income often take on volunteer work in addition to their regular jobs. Volunteering at a hospital, food bank, art museum, or school gives them a feeling of fulfillment and satisfaction for having a positive effect on their community. This, in turn, makes their "day job" more bearable because they're not depending on it for 100% of their work happiness.

You may wonder: Won't working longer hours with two jobs lead to burnout? Not necessarily. The risk of burnout is more a factor of how you *feel* about your job rather than how many hours you work at it.

Years ago, I had a friend who got a job as a telemarketer. The job required him to cold-call businesspeople at work and try to sell them various business services. He was paid by the hour and on commission. The more calls he made and the more products he sold, the more money he made. Each shift was four hours long. That was it: just four hours. In those four hours, he made as many as 200 phone calls to complete strangers. The manager walked around the call center, making sure everyone was on the phone. The work was mentally exhausting, and at the end of the shift, my friend said he felt like he had gone a couple of rounds with Mike Tyson.

At the end of four hours, he had the option to sign up for another four-hour shift. He never did. Out of 30 or so people in the call center, no more than two or three "hard core" salespeople ever took a second shift. For those two or three, something about the work didn't bother them. They actually *liked* it. They *thrived* on it. Everyone else, including my friend, couldn't wait to get out of there.

It's not the hours you work that matter so much as how you feel during those hours. If you do your time at your regular job and then spend a few hours doing something you really love, your "happy fuel tank" will be refilled, making it easier to repeat the process the next day.

KNOW YOUR DESIRED FUTURE STATE

If developing a side gig is not what you want to do, and you're thoroughly unhappy in your current job and industry, you should consider a new line of work. A total makeover. Something that will open the door to working happy with a satisfying work/life synergy that will last a long time.

To make such a change, it's important that you know yourself and what you affirmatively *want* to do. I'll explain. It's one thing to know what you don't like and what makes you burned out. Knowing where you've been and where you are now is necessary and valuable, but if you want to improve your life, you need to have a *desired future state* in mind. You need to be able to envision the career you want. This career may be something that you've had in the back of your mind for years but never thought possible, or a new opportunity that didn't exist until now. Whatever it is, it's something that makes you say, "Hey, I could do that!"

This is important for some very practical reasons. Unless you're wealthy and can afford to do nothing, you need to support yourself. Your *present state* is that you have a job that pays the bills. You may hate your job, but you probably can't afford to just walk away from it. Remember, all states have a federal/state unemployment insurance program, but in most states, it's only available if you are separated from your job through no fault of your own. This means your company has to lay you off or otherwise eliminate your job through downsizing or seasonal cutbacks. If this happens to you, you can collect unemployment benefits, which can make a big difference while you hunt for another job. But you cannot just walk away from your job or quit. If you do that, you probably won't qualify for benefits. You'll be on your own to pay the rent while you look for another opportunity.

This is why the ironclad advice that every career counselor gives is: *Don't quit your job until you've been hired by another company.* Don't act rashly. Keep in mind your long-term goal, which is to achieve your desired future on your terms. Hold onto your present position while you look for another. Make sure you use your own time and resources to conduct your search; to do it on company time would be unethical.

To transition from your present state of working unhappy to a future state of working happy with work/life synergy, you need to plan carefully.

LOOK AT THE BIG PICTURE

Let's take a step back and look at the problem in its entirety.

You probably started working a summer job when you were in high school or college. Unless you were already interested in a particular career path, like Bill Gates or grocer Tom Bonesho, you probably had no clear idea of what type of job you wanted.

The nice thing is that when you're living at home and you need to get a summer job because your parents want you to stay out of trouble and make some money so they can stop giving you an allowance, you have the luxury of taking any job that comes along. It doesn't matter if you hate it; you'll be quitting in August anyway. As long as the job isn't truly horrible, you'll do just about anything.

Kids will tell you all kinds of stories about their summer jobs. One son of a family friend landed a job on the overnight shift at a donut shop. He worked from 8:00 p.m. until 4:00 a.m. making fresh donuts for the next day. He learned all about making donuts. The following summer his dad got him a job at a foundry where they made industrial bronze and aluminum castings. The hours for this job were 7:00 a.m. until 3:00 p.m.

The kid had zero interest in making a career out of either donuts or industrial castings, but surprisingly, he treasured the experiences.

Neither job was permanent, which meant that he was working happy each summer. These jobs showed him a side of life that he was unlikely to have seen and would probably never see again. They were not unlike spending a summer studying abroad, except they were close to home and provided a paycheck.

Comedian and former *Tonight Show* host Jay Leno has spoken fondly about the summer he spent working at a McDonald's restaurant in his hometown of Andover, Massachusetts. He told this story to author Cody Teets in *Golden Opportunity: Remarkable Careers That Began at McDonald's:*

One morning, while preparing to make a batch of French fries, Leno walked into the restaurant's storage room to pick up a supply of potatoes. Tom Curtin, the owner-operator, was with him. They noticed something peculiar: Resting on top of the sack of potatoes was a pair of underpants.

"Sometimes crew members changed into their uniforms at work, and somebody had apparently forgotten their underpants," Leno said. "I expected Tom to tell me to throw out the top layer of potatoes and wash the rest. Instead, he said simply, 'Get rid of all those potatoes. Get rid of that whole batch. Just get rid of all of it.'"

Leno was impressed that Tom Curtin took no chances. "The standards for quality were quite high," Leno shared. "It was one of those life lessons I never forgot."[46]

When you take a summer job as a kid, it doesn't matter what you want for a career. In fact, it's probably beneficial that you take an odd job so that you experience what you typically would never be exposed to, get yourself out of your comfort zone, and learn basic work skills such as punctuality, professionalism, and job behavior.

As you get older, the stakes get higher. You have rent or a mortgage to pay and perhaps a family to support. You're no longer taking random summer jobs; you need to build a serious career.

But here's the million-dollar question: What if you don't know what will make you happy? What if you try but cannot envision your desired future?

If you're an adult with financial responsibilities, you can't just pretend you're a kid looking for a summer job and ready to try anything. You have too much to lose with that type of gamble.

No, you need to figure out what will make you happy.

The important questions you need to resolve are these: What is your desired future state? Where do you want to be in a year, five years, or 10 years? What do you see yourself doing?

To answer these questions, you may benefit from professional career counseling. Typically, a career counselor will interview you and have you take a series of tests to determine your affinity for various career paths. Such tests may include the Myers-Briggs Type Indicator (discussed in the following chapter), Who Am I?, The Self-Directed Search, Pymetrics, Career Strengths Test, and others.

These tests will help you zero in on two things:

1. The skills you have to offer.
2. The things you like to do.

Ideally, these two things should be in alignment. For example, if you have skills in financial accounting and you happen to enjoy it, then it's a no-brainer that you should probably look for a career in that area. In your present job, you may feel like your skills are being wasted or underutilized, and this imbalance could be the root of your unhappiness.

The formula is this: Your skills + Your enjoyment = Working happy.

It's very possible that you have professional training or skills in an industry for which you now have no interest. Don't stay in a job because you know how to do it and do it well. You have to have the second part of the equation, "your enjoyment," in order to work happy. A loss of enjoyment can occur because people change. Don't feel guilty if you have evolved!

MONEY AND TRAINING

There are two big things that keep people trapped in jobs and careers they don't like: money and training.

Transitioning to a new career can mean a loss of income, either because you're not working for a while or because you would be taking a significant pay cut in order to enter a new industry. The solution to this is to plan ahead.

As you contemplate your future state with a new career, you'll need to crunch the numbers. You'll need to estimate how long it will take you to use up any severance package or unemployment insurance funds you may receive, how long your savings may last, and when you think you'll be able to activate your income stream again with a new job. You may also think about cutting your expenses and selling your boat or vacation home. These are questions that only you can answer.

One thing to remember is that if you hated your job, you may have compensated for that dislike by buying toys and goodies to make yourself happy. If you find a career where you'll be working happy and enjoying a good work/life synergy, it's certain those expensive toys will be much less necessary. You might not even miss them when they're gone.

As for training, you may need to go back to school for another degree or get certification training. The training required to enter a new career may take anywhere from just a few weeks to many years. For example, if you decide you want to become a lawyer, in most states, you'll need to get your bachelor of arts degree (if you haven't already), take the Law School Admission Test (LSAT) or Graduate Record Examinations (GRE), go to law school to earn your juris doctor degree (three years full time, up to five years part-time), and pass the bar exam in your state.

If you want to enter the healthcare industry, the easiest portal of entry is to become certified for one of many entry-level positions, including phlebotomy, cardiac technician, medical assistant, and others. Such training typically takes a few months.

Career training can be a significant expense, and you may need to investigate financing. If you work for a large company, the first place you should look to is your employer. Many companies offer subsidies or outright full tuition for learning programs, even master's degree programs, that relate to the company's business activities and make you a more valuable employee. Going back to school at the company's expense can have the double benefit of giving you training at a low cost and — just maybe — making your present workplace more attractive and less likely to give you burnout. It could be a win-win for both parties.

Remember, though, that if your employer sends you to school, the company will almost certainly require you to sign a commitment letter stating you'll stay with the company for a specified number of years. If you go to school on the company's dime and then quit, that's not very nice, and you may be liable for the tuition bill. Continuing education is an investment your employer makes in you, and you should accept it knowing that you'll honor your commitment to the company.

If your employer doesn't offer training, you can pay for it by getting a student loan.

The good news is that many reputable colleges offer online courses that are inexpensive and count toward a degree or certification.

No matter how you do it, you can keep working at your present job that you dislike while training for a new career. And here's the amazing part: When you put your plan into action, your present job will suddenly become more bearable because, like the kid working as a donut fryer in the summer, you'll see the light at the end of the tunnel. Your dreary work will now have a positive purpose. You'll clearly see your desired future state, and you may even know the date of its arrival.

AN UNSATISFIED AFFINITY: THE CAREER JOURNEY OF VERA WANG

As we've mentioned, Americans are estimated to change careers an average of four times during their life. Some people stick with just one career, while others are more mobile, like working vagabonds journeying from industry to industry.

In all of this fluidity, it's safe to say that most people who change careers make lateral shifts into another industry that has some connection with what they've been trained to do. For example, you don't see many fast-food company executives suddenly become airline executives because the skill sets are just too different; however, you might very well see someone in the fast-food industry shift to hospitality or to supermarkets because there are many skills in common.

Most people seeking work/life synergy shift into industries for which they have an *unsatisfied affinity*. By that, I mean the person has a feeling or intuition about what they want in life and in their career, but for whatever reason, they're not pursuing it.

Vera Wang, the renowned fashion designer, made the change. Wang was born June 27, 1949, in New York City. Her mother worked as a translator for the United Nations, and her father owned a prosperous medicine company. The family was affluent, and at age eight, Vera began training as a figure skater. She was usually on the ice by 6:00 a.m. so she could practice before school, and her day often ended with more practice. She competed at the 1968 U.S. Figure Skating Championships and that same year was presented as a debutante to high society at the International Debutante Ball at the Waldorf Astoria in New York City.

But then she failed to qualify for the U.S. Olympic skating team at the 1968 games in Grenoble, France. As she told Olympics.com, "I had a nervous breakdown and ended up doing a semester in Paris." She added, "It was in the French capital where I realized I had a passion for fashion."[47]

She studied at the University of Paris before completing her degree in art history at Sarah Lawrence College. Immediately upon graduation in 1971, she got a huge break: *Vogue* magazine hired her to be an assistant to the fashion director. She quickly moved up in the company, becoming fashion editor at age 23, responsible for the magazine's editorial fashion spreads. The job was demanding and left little time for her to pursue her dream of designing. She stayed at *Vogue* for 17 years, but after being turned down for the editor-in-chief position, she left in 1987 to join Ralph Lauren, for whom she designed accessories for the fashion label.

Two years later, she was engaged to be married, but she had a problem: She didn't like any of the wedding dresses she saw in the bridal shops. She told Jane Sharp of *Biography Magazine*, "I wanted something more elegant and subdued, but there wasn't anything. I realized the desire to fill that niche." She decided to create her own dress. She sketched the design and commissioned a dressmaker to tailor the elaborate gown at a cost of $10,000.[48]

Bolstered by the feeling of confidence in her first step as a designer of her own wedding dress, at age 40, she resigned from Ralph Lauren. With financial backing from her father, Wang opened her own bridal boutique, Vera Wang Bridal House, in the upscale Carlyle Hotel on Madison Avenue in New York City.

Despite her success as an employee at prestigious companies, she had insecurities about becoming an entrepreneur. As she told *Harvard Business Review* in 2019, "Perhaps I would have preferred to start off at age 20 or 30, but I don't think I would have been anywhere near equipped to know what it takes to be in business. Even at 40, I wasn't entirely sure I should be doing it. It wasn't an era for start-ups. I'd always felt I should learn and earn, and I'd already had two incredible careers working for others — at Condé Nast and then Ralph Lauren — the best in the industry. Still, I didn't feel very qualified or secure. I never thought I deserved to found a company.... I didn't know anything about dress design. I didn't feel ready. And when I left Ralph, a lot of doors that had been open to me slammed shut, whether it was a fabric manufacturer or a party I wanted to go to, because I was now so small. Harsh. But my DNA was to find something I felt passionate about, to make a difference, and to work, so that's what I did."[49]

Have you ever felt this way: hesitant and insecure, yet having a strong feeling that you should be following the path dictated by your heart? Maybe now is the time to respond to that feeling!

In the brutally competitive bridal wear industry, Vera Wang persisted. At first, she sold couture gowns by designers Guy Laroche, Arnold Scali, Carolina Herrera, and Christian Dior, but then began offering her own designs. They proved so popular that before long, the store sold her creations exclusively. Wang expanded her collection to include bridesmaids' dresses and couture evening gowns.

I'm just guessing, but I'll bet that when she first opened her own bridal boutique, she worked longer and harder than she ever had before, but because she was working happy and with powerful work/life synergy, she felt good about herself and her life.

Wang never forgot her love for figure skating, and in 1992 and 1994, figure skater Nancy Kerrigan generated global attention wearing Wang designs at the Winter Olympics. Wang went on to create costumes for other Olympic skaters, including Nathan Chen and Michelle Kwan. Soon, actresses and celebrities were wearing her creations on television and at highly publicized events.

In the 21st century, Wang continued to expand her global brand; she offered her first ready-to-wear collection, opened wedding gown boutiques in the United States, and sold her designs through high-end retailers around the world. Wang launched a fragrance, published a highly acclaimed wedding guide, and expanded her business to include lingerie, jewelry, home products, and even desserts.

In 2018, Wang ranked 34th in Forbes' list of America's Richest Self-Made Women, and her revenues reached $630 million that year. She's still most well known as a designer of wedding dresses and has designed them for Mariah Carey, Chelsea Clinton, Alicia Keys, Ivanka Trump, Khloe and Kim Kardashian, Hilary Duff, Victoria Beckham, and many others.

Vera Wang is someone who made important transitions in her life, with each transition bringing her closer to her goal of making people feel good about themselves by being beautifully dressed. Her career journey began as a figure skater, but something inside her told her that although she had extensive training as a skater and her family's support, it was not to be her calling in life.

Her failure to qualify for the Olympics was, to her, a message from the universe that she needed to change. But she didn't yet see herself as a fashion designer — the reality seemed beyond her reach. She knew she had an affinity for fashion design, but since she didn't know how to make it a part of her own life, she entered the fashion magazine publishing business, which brought her a step closer to her calling, but it was still not exactly what she was born to do. She may have stayed in the publishing industry had she not been passed over for the job of editor-in-chief at *Vogue*. That event was the second message to her, and her next job, being an accessories designer for Ralph Lauren, brought her one more step closer to what she needed to be.

But she wasn't there yet! There was one more message from the universe coming: When she went shopping for a wedding dress for herself and couldn't find what she wanted, she realized that her true calling was to help other brides have beautiful and romantic weddings, starting with the dress. This realization and her growing confidence, as well as financial and spiritual encouragement from her father, were the keys to unleashing her full potential and allowing her to develop her full capabilities as an artist, businessperson, and human being.

It's common for people to have unsatisfied affinities — that is, a yearning for an activity or vocation that's not the focus of their work life. The question is, if you have such a feeling, to what extent should you act on it and even try to make it your career?

Let's say you're a company executive, and your hobby is flyfishing. In fact, you're an expert at freshwater flyfishing, and you often give advice to others about how to get started in the sport and where to go for the best fishing.

Your corporate job pays $200,000 a year. At the moment, you figure your flyfishing hobby *costs* you $10,000 a year. And yet, deep down inside, you find yourself identifying less and less with the corporate world and more and more with the wilderness. At your desk in the office, you wish you were on the way to your secret fishing hole, and while you're waist-deep in a cold mountain stream, you wish you never had to go back to the city.

If this sounds familiar, only you can decide what you want to do — or *should* do.

Look at the possibilities. Is there a way you could make money with your passion for flyfishing? Can you become a tour guide, or produce films about fishing, or run a fishing resort? What services can you provide that will bring you the income you need?

Look at your responsibilities. Do you have a spouse and children? Could you change careers and downsize your income without harming those who depend on you?

If you cannot leave your corporate job, can you scale it back to allow more time for fishing?

You have an income now. Can you divert some of it to invest in a fishing resort in the mountains, and when you have a big enough stake in that enterprise, switch careers and make it a full-time job?

When Vera Wang launched her bridal shop, she was very lucky to have her father's financial support and business expertise, but at the end of the day, it was her vision and determination that made it a success. If you have an unsatisfied affinity, there's no reason to ignore it. Celebrate it and try to find a way to incorporate it into your life of working happy.

Fargo during the faked sales scandal. Some leaders, like the late Jack Welch at General Electric, enjoy creating a "fight-or-flight" culture in their company. In his case, the purported reason was to "keep people on their toes" because everyone knew the bottom performers would be fired.

3. If you stay in a fight-or-flight mode for a prolonged period of time, the sustained stress to your mind and body will be damaging. Overexposure to cortisol and other stress hormones will disrupt many of your body's natural processes, putting you at increased risk of many health problems. For example, cortisol increases appetite, so you'll want to eat more to obtain extra energy. It also increases the storage of unused nutrients as fat.

   There are many others:
   - Anxiety
   - Depression
   - Digestive problems
   - Headaches
   - Heart disease, heart attack, high blood pressure, and stroke
   - Memory and concentration impairment
   - Muscle pain and tension
   - Sleep problems
   - Weight gain

When building your work/life synergy, obviously the very last thing you want or need is to be under prolonged stress. It's unpleasant, and it's bad for your health. But here's the thing: Only you can decide what's stressful for you.

Some people thrive on competition at work, such as people in sales. Some people, such as sports figures or high-rise steelworkers, enjoy physically challenging jobs. Librarians need peace and tranquility. Elementary school teachers enjoy the energy of children, even though they may be driven by rambunctious kids to play a game of "hide and no seek."

Your emotional resilience is yours alone, and you owe it to yourself to find the role in which you feel comfortable, regardless of what anyone else thinks.

With deliberate consciousness and practice, you can strengthen your emotional resilience. With the right tools, you can become more resilient, even if you are naturally more sensitive to the slings and arrows that people and life throw at you.

Here are some traits of emotional resilience that you can develop in yourself.

OPTIMISM

"Dispositional optimism" is defined as the generalized, relatively stable tendency to expect good outcomes across important life domains. If you're optimistic, you believe that success is possible and good things will happen as a result of your hard work. The future is bright, and you feel good about your life. You recognize the positive aspects in challenging situations and believe in their strength. You understand the words of Thomas Edison, who, just before he found success with the light bulb, said, "I have not failed. I've just found 10,000 ways that won't work."

Being optimistic is foundational to achieving work/life synergy. You need to believe that your future is bright and you have something to live for — your vocation, your family, your community. This is perhaps the reason immigrants tend to have high levels of optimism: They're generally leaving a dismal present in search of a better future.

According to a survey by Western Union, migrants are extremely optimistic about their economic and social prospects in their new countries. Fully 86% of people who had recently immigrated to the United States said they viewed their adopted country positively. Ninety-five percent of U.S. migrants agreed that they could do well if they worked hard. By a large majority, migrants reported greater levels of optimism and success than their native-born counterparts.

In every country surveyed, immigrants reported that the top reason for emigrating to the new country was better job prospects, followed by higher income, education, and training.[50]

Optimism will not only lower your likelihood of burnout, but it may help you live longer. A number of studies have shown that optimists enjoy lower levels of stress, higher levels of well-being, better sleep, and better cardiovascular health and immune function.

A groundbreaking 2019 study based on data from the 69,744 women from the Nurses' Health Study (NHS) and 1,429 men from the Veterans Affairs (VA) Normative Aging Study (NAS) found that women in the highest versus lowest optimism quartile had 14.9% longer life span. Optimistic men performed similarly. Participants with the highest versus lowest optimism levels had 1.5 (women) and 1.7 (men) greater odds of surviving to age 85.[51]

These findings are especially impressive because the results remained even after accounting for other factors known to predict a long life, such as education level, economic status, ethnicity, and mental or physical health.

One more thing to think about: Your level of optimism can change over the course of your life. Researchers have found that optimism tends to increase across younger adulthood, level off in midlife, and then decline in older adulthood. This is most likely the result of how we view ourselves and the world as we pass through life with its various successes and setbacks.

We experience changes in goals, expectations, social networks, and, of course, our own biological and physical systems. People who receive a challenging health diagnosis may become less optimistic, particularly if they're told that a chronic illness could shorten their life or bring severe physical limitations or pain. Conversely, people who are getting married might see an increase in optimism because they look forward to sharing positive life experiences with a person they love.[52]

Any discussion of optimism should touch upon the so-called law of attraction. Its more radical adherents assert that if you think about a new car, you will have one. Just like that! This is a bit silly, but the truth embodied in the law of attraction is this: If you *believe* good things will happen to you, you're more likely to *make them* happen for yourself.

If you interview for a new job and you believe you can get it, your positivity will make it more likely to happen. If you don't believe you can get it, then you're likely to get exactly what you expect, which is nothing. People who believe good things are coming their way are more likely to recognize a good thing and seize upon it. People who expect bad things are more likely to find them. This is the true law of attraction.

EMOTIONAL INTELLIGENCE

Emotional intelligence (EI) is a set of skills that help you recognize, understand, and manage your own emotions as well as recognize, understand, and influence the emotions of others. Critical in building and maintaining personal relationships as well as in influencing others, EI will help you throughout your career and wherever you dwell in an organizational structure.

You probably know one or more people who seem emotionally oblivious in the sense they have strong feelings, even anger, without having a reason they can clearly articulate. They also do or say things that hurt other people without realizing what they've done. In contrast, people with emotional intelligence or awareness understand what they're feeling and why. Because they're more in touch with their own inner life, they can better empathize with the feelings of others.

This type of emotional understanding allows you to respond appropriately when others cross the line and better regulate and cope when you feel attacked and are tempted to strike back. Remember that you have no control over what other people do, but you can control what you do.

Also, it's good to remember that if someone on the job is mean or rude to you, there's a 99% likelihood they're mean or rude to other people as well. Of course, they're not rude to the boss; many mean people are sugar-sweet to their superiors. In other words, it may not be just you; this person is likely a jerk to everyone. Don't take it personally.

As described by Daniel Golman, author of the bestselling book *Emotional Intelligence*, EI has four main components.

1. Self-Awareness

If you don't understand yourself, understanding other people will be difficult. Your emotions, which you have every waking moment, impact your mood, performance, behaviors, and interactions with other people. If you're self-aware, you tend to be more confident and more creative, and you communicate more effectively, make better decisions, and build stronger relationships.

If you feel as though your self-awareness is low, you can take any one of a number of self-administered personality tests. There's an entire industry devoted to these tests that purport to tell you what type of person you are and, perhaps most usefully, what type of career you might be suited for. Many of them are free, but many are spurious or just "click bait" designed to harvest your personal info. I'd stick with the major brands.

The Myers-Briggs Type Indicator (MBTI) is one of the most popular self-assessment tools. Created by Katharine Cook Briggs and her daughter, Isabel Briggs Myers, it's an introspective self-report questionnaire indicating differing psychological preferences in how you perceive the world. It's based on Carl Jung's theory, which posited four principal psychological functions by which humans experience the world: sensation, intuition, feeling, and thinking.

In the MBTI universe, there are four pairs of personality categories or "dichotomies": introversion/extraversion, sensing/intuition, thinking/feeling, and judging/perceiving. Each person is said to have one preferred quality from each category, producing 16 unique types.

According to the MBTI system, you combine your preferences to arrive at your personality type. The 16 types are referred to by an abbreviation of the initial letters of each of the four type preferences. Each of the 16 personality types has a name. For example, the acronym ISTP would denote introversion, sensing, thinking, and perceiving. This person is known as The Crafter. He or she is fearless and independent, loves adventure and new experiences, but is not well-attuned to the emotional states of others, sometimes coming across as insensitive or stoic, and are results-oriented.

(To avoid confusion, the dichotomy "intuition" is denoted not with an "I" but with an "N.")

There is no "score" that's higher or lower than any other. There is no combination considered "better" or "worse" than another; all types are viewed as equally human and valuable. The key is to find the right vocation that suits your personality type.

For example, if your type is ISTP, the qualities of introversion, sensing, thinking, and perceiving might not be what you'd need to be a commissioned salesperson. On the other hand, if your type is EFNJ (The Protagonist), the qualities of extraversion, feeling, intuition, and judging might serve you very well as a commissioned salesperson. Of course, this is not scientific, and every person is different, but such a test can give you something to think about.

The DiSC Assessment was designed to measure dominance, influence, steadiness, and conscientiousness. Introduced by Walter Clark in 1940, the questionnaire was created predominantly for organizational use and can be used for leadership and executive development, conflict management, communication, team building, management training, sales training, customer services, and job coaching.

DiSC is an acronym for the four main personality profiles described in the DiSC model: (D)ominance, (i)nfluence, (S)teadiness, and (C)onscientiousness.

People with D personalities tend to be confident and place an emphasis on accomplishing bottom-line results.

People with i personalities tend to be more open and place emphasis on relationships and influencing or persuading others.

People with S personalities tend to be dependable and place an emphasis on cooperation and sincerity.

People with C personalities tend to place emphasis on quality, accuracy, expertise, and competency.

The company is careful to say that "no DiSC style is 'better' than any other, and we all use each of the four styles as we go about our daily lives. DiSC simply helps us find out which style we tend to gravitate toward most — our comfort zone."[53]

The DiSC assessment is designed to be easy to use, easy to administer, and to be delivered by anyone. The online test comprises 28 questions; for each question you pick a word you think is most like yourself and a word that is least like yourself. Prices for this assessment depend on the type of career tested, and the size and type of team being assessed.

There are many more such tests. You can even go to a website like Truity.com and take several tests to get an overall picture of what they say about you.

Ask yourself: Do you feel as though you know yourself well? This is a tricky question because most of us may think we know ourselves, but this belief gets intermingled with what we hope or imagine ourselves to be, as well as what we don't want to be. We inflate our positive attributes and reduce our shortcomings, or we do the opposite and magnify our faults while diminishing our skills. None of these personality tests can capture your entire personality, but they can offer you a fresh perspective on yourself.

2. Self-Management

This is your ability to regulate your emotions and behaviors. Once you're aware of your emotions, you can effectively manage them and keep the disruptive behaviors and impulses under control.

When you have strong self-management, and you're in a tense or stressful situation, you can pause and take a deep breath. This will help you to be calm and think before you speak or act.

Self-managed people tend to have a positive outlook and are adaptable to a variety of situations and circumstances. Emotions can be contagious, just like a lack of self-regulation and negativity can be. Those who cannot contain their negative emotions and impulses often set off a chain reaction of negative emotions in others, which increases feelings of burnout.

Ask yourself: Do you sometimes "fly off the handle" or overreact and regret it later? Many people have emotional "triggers" that are like your funny bone — the slightest tap sends a shooting pain into your body. Such triggers often have their roots in a childhood or adult trauma that you may want to investigate with a professional.

Also, if you are in an unfamiliar situation, you're more likely to feel panicked or out of control. This is perfectly natural. The first time you make a presentation in front of a large audience, you may feel tense, clammy, and even afraid. That's because it's new to you.

But if you do it again and again, it will become second nature, and you may even enjoy it.

3. Social Awareness

This is pretty much what it sounds like: our ability to "read" and understand the emotions of others. It's about taking the focus off us and thinking about those around us. This isn't always easy, especially if we're wrapped up in our work and consumed by our own thoughts.

A key component of social awareness is empathy, which is identifying what others feel, understanding the emotion, and wishing to improve their experience. It's not about how *you* would feel in their situation, but rather, how *they actually feel*. This is an important distinction. For example, someone who was born and raised in their hometown cannot be expected to know exactly how a recent immigrant feels, but with social awareness, they can empathize with that person's situation.

People with strong social awareness tend to be kind. True kindness may include giving others difficult feedback, and socially aware people are good at delivering "tough love" because they understand the other person and want to help them do better.

It's also about consideration for others and knowing how the things we do and say affect them. If you bring a big box of donuts to the office and pass them around knowing full well that some of your colleagues are diabetic and need to avoid sugar, you're not exhibiting good social awareness.

Ask yourself: Are you ever caught off guard by someone's response to you? When you talk about your favorite political candidate or express your personal religious views, do some people look away? That's probably because they have differing views and don't want to engage with you. You wouldn't like it if a colleague came to work and started spouting off some personal ideology that you find repugnant. Be aware and be discreet!

4. Relationship Management

In the business world, relationship management means maintaining good and positive connections between an organization and its customers. In life, it goes further and means managing and maintaining positive relationships with everyone: your family, community, colleagues, and friends.

Relationship management is the art of influencing people to become the best version of themselves. An effective influencer has robust interpersonal skills, which can be learned and taught. The better you get at these skills, the better you will be able to manage your relationships at work and at home.

The goal is to reduce friction and maximize happiness. Friction, in the form of misunderstandings and conflict, is a prime source of burnout, and the more you can lower it, the better. This leads to greater mutual happiness, which is also an antidote to burnout.

Ask yourself: Why should you conform? You've probably heard the expression, "When in Rome, do as the Romans do." This means that you should try to respect and observe the customs and habits of the people around you, whether in Rome or your own hometown. If you're self-centered, you might reply, "Why should I conform to them? They can just as well conform to me." It may seem paradoxical, but if you understand them and can blend in with them, you'll have more influence and more authority because you'll be breaking down barriers. Your confidence will show, and the people around you will be flattered.

INTERNAL LOCUS OF CONTROL

To achieve true emotional resilience, you must be in control of your thoughts and emotions, even when life is not going your way.

What we're talking about is the concept of *psychological* free will. To clarify, I am not talking about the metaphysical subject of whether you believe in free will versus fatalism or determinism. We all know people on both sides of this debate and some who are in between.

What I am getting at is that when you drill down more deeply, you can see that many people allow the outside world — a task at work, what a colleague says, a bad break, whatever — to be in control of how they think and how they feel. They become like a leaf in the wind, blown this way and that, and their actions begin to reflect their thoughts and become more haphazard. Ultimately, their state of mind rattles in constant anxiety.

While you cannot control the external world, you can control how you interact with it and how you feel about it. If you are never able to take responsibility for your psychological state of mind, you will never be able to take action to correct or influence a situation.

It is easy to feel victimized and just say to yourself, "It's not my fault. I'm just unlucky. It's a conspiracy against me. They are to blame, not me." It becomes an odd combination of proclaiming one's own incompetence while blaming the world for that incompetence.

When you harness your psychological process and take responsibility for your own thoughts and emotions, it can actually result in more freedom and more happiness. Remember the old Buddhist saying: "Pain is inevitable. Suffering is optional." A hurricane destroying your house is painful and out of your control, but the degree to which you will suffer is largely under your control. You can play the victim card, wallow in your misery, and complain about how life is unfair, or you can exert your locus of control, resolve to pick yourself up, and get your life back on track.

When you take control, you experience lower stress; with a strong internal locus of control, you aren't waiting fearfully for the next bad thing to happen. You know you can handle what life dishes out, and your realistic view of the world makes you more proactive in dealing with stressors in your life, more solution-oriented, and with a greater sense of inner control.

Ask yourself: Do you ruminate over the past and worry about the future? If so, you are likely losing your focus on the present.

Are you regularly stressed out at work? Don't reflexively blame your job! The receptionist and chief executive officer will both say they are stressed. Remember that while your job is *what you do*, it's not *who you are*. The root cause of your stress may be your inability to retain control of yourself, your thoughts, and your emotions. Your perceptions can become your reality.

Do you find that you are routinely the victim of circumstance or that you are waiting for that one thing to change in order for life to be better? You need to get control now. Remember that each phase of life presents its own challenges: As a toddler, just about anything sets you off. As a teenager, you were invincible but bewildered and absolutely sure that the adult world was your enemy. When we reach our middle age, in comes the mid-life crisis and running the rat race. And finally, in our old age, our body begins to decline while our minds stay active. Or vice versa. Problems will always persist and be easy to palpate. We need to think differently.

Globally, in the past few decades, billions of people have been lifted out of poverty. We have smart phones that carry vastly more computing power than the Apollo moon mission had, but gravity always seems to help us find fault in ourselves or others. With our outside world advancing in ways previous generations couldn't even conceive of, convenience can be created almost anywhere, but we can't confuse this condition with comfort or well-being.

HEDONIC AND EUDAIMONIC WELL-BEING

Looking to the outside world to give you comfort or inner wellness and to strengthen your inner locus is never sustainable. When you think about it, it makes no sense to assert the outside world can make you *happy* if you then *deny* it can make you *unhappy*. You can't have it both ways. It's a tricky balance because any reasonable person will say, "The birth of your child should make you happy. Getting the job you want should make you happy. Seeing your child graduate from college should make you happy." This is true. These achievements are good things and should produce good feelings, but your deep-down happiness should not *depend* on them.

Likewise, any reasonable person would say, "Seeing your child sick in bed should make you unhappy. Getting laid off from your job, through no fault of your own, should make you unhappy." Fair enough! These negative events can make you feel sad, but your vision of yourself as a fundamentally happy person shouldn't change.

The ancient Greeks addressed this issue, and in response, they defined two forms of happiness or well-being: *hedonic* and *eudaimonic*.

Aristippus (435–356 BCE) taught that your goal should be to experience the maximum amount of pleasure and that your happiness comprised the totality of your hedonic moments. Hedonic well-being refers to the pleasures or happiness that we derive from doing what we like or avoiding what we do not like. The most common examples of hedonic pleasure include food, sex, music, TV shows, funny cat videos, and other sensory activities. These pleasures are transitory, and once you stop experiencing them, they quickly fade.

In contrast, Aristotle (384–322 BCE) wrote in his *Nichomachean Ethics* that the highest of all human conditions is *eudaimonia*, which he defined as the behavior of the soul in accord with virtue. It's long-term personal excellence and exploring the best within us. It's produced when you achieve something meaningful, like graduating from college, working productively in a career with personal significance, or helping other people lead better lives.

You may ask, if eudaimonia is the superior form of well-being, are we, therefore, supposed to avoid all hedonistic pleasure? No, of course not. A life without brief sensory pleasures would be boring and dreary. Human beings need stimulation in all its forms, and many of these forms, such as laughter, have measurable health benefits. But no hedonistic pleasure can replace the deeper, longer-lasting satisfaction of eudaimonic achievements. They can only be attained when you have a strong internal locus of control and are consciously guiding your life and your emotions using your own inner strength.

Find strength within yourself; it costs you nothing and is endlessly renewable.

PERSEVERANCE

Perseverance refers to your ability to pursue a goal or passion over time and stick with it when you encounter obstacles or setbacks. Notice that I said "when" you encounter setbacks, not "if." In any worthwhile endeavor, setbacks are to be expected.

Earlier in the book, I mentioned Thomas Edison. For many people, he personifies perseverance; in fact, he's responsible for the statement, "Genius is 1% inspiration and 99% perspiration."

Edison is a fertile source of quotes; here's another: "Many of life's failures are people who did not realize how close they were to success when they gave up."

The stories about how he and his assistants tested thousands of substances when searching for the one that would work best in a light bulb are true. At the time, in the 1870s, the basic technology for making an electric light was well-understood by many scientists around the world. In fact, the first working electric light had been demonstrated in 1802 in England by Humphry Davy, who connected wires to his battery and a piece of carbon. The carbon glowed, producing light. His invention was known as the electric arc lamp. The problem? It didn't last long, and it was *too bright* for indoor use.

Starting in the 1870s, arc lighting was widely used for street and large building lighting. So the challenge Edison and the others faced was to produce a bulb that was dimmer than an arc light, cheap to produce, and whose filament would last a long time. For the filament, Edison finally settled on carbonized bamboo fiber, which lasted more than 1,200 hours.

"Before I got through," he recalled, "I tested no fewer than 6,000 vegetable growths and ransacked the world for the most suitable filament material.... The electric light has caused me the greatest amount of study and has required the most elaborate experiments. I was never myself discouraged or inclined to be hopeless of success. I cannot say the same for all my associates."[54]

How could Edison have shown such perseverance? Simple: He loved every minute of his work. He enjoyed true work/life synergy.

SENSE OF HUMOR

To get started on this topic, let's consider a quote from President Dwight D. Eisenhower: "A sense of humor is part of the art of leadership, of getting along with people, of getting things done."

How true! Leaders who know how to keep the mood light even when the work is hard have more productive employees. But why is that? What is it about expressing and sharing levity that makes life more fun, or at least more bearable, and can actually help us work harder?

There really is some truth and science behind the phrase, "Laughter is the best medicine." Aside from being a pleasant diversion for your thoughts, when you're laughing at a co-worker's joke, you're temporarily distracted from the stress of your job. Laughter's proven physiological benefits include:

Stimulates key organs. Laughter increases the endorphins released by your brain, boosts your intake of oxygen-rich air, and stimulates your heart, lungs, and muscles. It exercises your diaphragm and enables you to take in more oxygenated air.

Relieves tension. Laughter can stimulate circulation and aid muscle relaxation, both of which can alleviate some of the physical symptoms of stress. It has been shown to improve your pain threshold, likely due to an endorphin-mediated opiate effect.

A robust laugh leads to a cascade of events that decrease the stress hormones that tax your immune system and give you that good, relaxed feeling.

Keeps you healthy. Laughter helps to boost the immune system, which makes you more resistant to disease. It does this by actually increasing the antibody-producing cells and T cells in your body, which are your primary defense agents against illness.

Helps quell emotional eating. When you laugh, it triggers the release of feel-good neurotransmitters. Even a friendly smile can trick your brain into thinking you're happy, reducing the need to eat to soothe your nerves or anxiety. Think about it this way: If you go to the movies and see a side-splitting comedy, how much popcorn are you going to eat? Now think about seeing a horror film. I'll bet you'll wolf down much more popcorn and snacks during the scary movie.

Gives you a new perspective. When you have emotional resilience, you can more easily laugh at life's difficulties. This helps put problems into perspective and shifts your viewpoint from seeing challenges as threats to seeing them as opportunities. This can alter how your body reacts to stress; the jolt of hormones that accompanies a fear response, if repeated often enough, can be damaging. After a good round of laughing, you may discover a new perspective on a problem. You might realize that you've gotten through other difficult periods and will get through this one, too.

Reduces tension by deflecting negativity. In the workplace, a sense of humor is a useful and important personal characteristic. Let's say, for example, you have a colleague whom you call Mr. Grumpy. He's just a big grouch with very little to say that's positive. While you must be respectful when you're in his presence, his thinly veiled insults could hurt you — but only if you let them. If you don't take them personally and instead view them as a symptom of his deep-rooted unhappiness, you'll be in a much stronger and more stable position. You can even find humor in the situation while feeling empathy for Mr. Grumpy.

WILLINGNESS TO FACE YOUR FEARS

If you want to reduce the power that something scary has over you, the solution is not to avoid it but to face it. Nowhere is this truer than at work. Think about what you're most afraid of in your workplace. I'll bet it's asking your boss for a raise. In second place is probably asking your boss to help you with a personal problem, such as a co-worker who's being abusive. You envision the scene: With a trembling hand, you knock on your boss's office door. "Come in," she says. You open the door. You wonder, do I look nervous? Can she see me sweating?

Your boss looks up. "Yes, what do you want?"

"Uhh, can we talk about something?"

Your boss glances at her watch to let you know her time is valuable. "Sure," she says. "Close the door. Have a seat."

And so on.

What can you do about this? Two things.

First, you can engage in low-stakes communications before the big meeting. Email your boss and ask if you can meet. Tell her why. Start with baby steps and proceed only if she's receptive. This will lower the stress level.

Second, tell yourself that the scary task will be a good experience and you'll learn from it. This is particularly effective if you're asked to speak in public and you're not a confident orator. Just say to yourself, "I'm not going to die up there. I should be grateful to have this learning experience. Yes, I will be terrible. But that's okay! I'll get better the more I do it." Lower your expectations and put a smile on your face. After all, you only live once — why not have many rich experiences?

The fact is that we are often hurt by our own sense of exaggerated fear and imagined disasters. We think the worst, but the reality is often nothing like what we imagined it to be. I'm reminded of my son, who thought there was a monster under the bed. But just like his father before him, he grew up and learned his fears were unfounded, and there was no monster under the bed.

We all suffer from our own imagination at times, usually when we're entering an unfamiliar situation for the first time — accepting a new job and having a new boss, being asked to deliver a speech to a large group, traveling to a foreign country on business, or assuming management over a team of people who used to be your peers. Persistently entertaining unfounded fears can quickly make working less happy and hasten burnout.

Ask yourself: Do you take everything super-seriously, or are you able to step back and smile at it all? If someone offends you, do you stew over it, or do you brush it off and chalk it up to the cost of being human? And if someone is aggressive or otherwise insecure, are you able to defuse the situation with a bit of humor? If you can, then this attribute will take you far in life.

REST AND RECOVER

Working happy with emotional resilience means that you find enjoyment in what you do, feel a sense of fulfillment for a job well done, and are not easily deterred by a setback. But human beings have limits, even when we're doing something we love. The body and brain both need time to recharge after a day of work, which is why we have the gift of sleep. This provides us with a 24-hour cycle of work and rest.

Sleep is extremely important for our health, and this has been repeatedly proven by research studies in which humans are deprived of sleep with consistently unhealthy results. When the brain is sleep-deprived, negative effects are reflected in alertness, vigilance, and simple attention; altered emotional functioning; and learning and memory. Other observed clinical effects were increased objective sleepiness; microsleeps, sometimes lasting just a few seconds but which can be disastrous when driving a car or operating machinery; decreased psychomotor performance on tasks involving short-term memory, reaction time, or vigilance; and degraded mood.

Volunteers who have willfully stayed awake for days at a time may experience microsleeps and hallucinations in which the brain, although technically awake, enters the REM dream cycle.

The hard-charging boss who brags about needing only four hours of sleep a night may find themselves experiencing elevated hypertension, higher heart rate, and a greater risk of fatal cardiovascular problems, such as heart attacks and stroke. Evidence suggests a lack of sleep may cause inflammation, which makes a blood clot more likely and disrupts the parts of the brain that control the circulatory system.

It's also related to elevated levels of cortisol, a stress hormone, as well as ghrelin, which can actually make people feel hungrier. Tiredness can lead to unhealthy cravings and overindulgence, leading to obesity and a decrease in stamina and physical activity.

To protect your emotional resilience, get enough sleep.

Since ancient times, people have recognized that in addition to the 24-hour cycle of work and sleep, we all need a full day of rest on a regular basis. By the word "rest" we mean some leisurely activity that is *not* the work you do the other six days of the week, even if you love it and have a good work/life synergy. The belief in a day of rest was established as early as the Old Testament, which told us that God created the world in six days and rested on the seventh. This report conveniently dovetailed with the fact that there are seven days in a week and 52 weeks in a year, so the weekly cycle could continue indefinitely.

Leonardo da Vinci, one of the greatest overachievers in human history, said, "Every now and then go away, have a little relaxation, for when you come back to your work, your judgment will be surer."

He meant that when you work hard on a project, you can become too close to it and lose your objectivity. By stepping away for a day and then coming back to it, you will have forgotten about it, and you'll see it fresh, as if for the first time. Defects to which you had become inured will suddenly seem glaring. You'll think, "Gee, why didn't I see that before?"

Speaking of Leonardo da Vinci, it may interest you to know that he painted the *Mona Lisa* — generally regarded as one of the most perfect works of art ever created — over a period of at least 16 years. (No one's exactly sure when he started it, but he was still fussing with it when he died in 1519.) He'd work on it for a while, put it aside, work on it again, and so on, year after year. This allowed him to become detached from it and see it objectively, without placing undeserved weight on one part or another.

Taking dedicated time for non-work will encourage you to have an identity distinct from your occupation, help you foster relationships beyond your fellow employees, and give you time to develop other activities and hobbies. Rather than defining your life by what you *do*, you'll begin to define it by who you *are*.

TAKE A TIME OUT

If the pace of work is rapid and the stakes are high, taking time out to step back and review the situation can be a smart idea that keeps you on your toes and better engaged in your work.

For example, in the medical field, any time we cut into a living body, the stakes are high. When we're preparing to perform a surgical procedure on a patient, before we make the first incision, we do a *time-out* — that's what it's called. During this important pause, we complete a checklist. We verify the patient's name, the exact location of the surgery (right or left), and the procedure that we are about to perform (remove gallstone or gallbladder, for example). Lastly, we always ask if the consent form has been signed.

A time-out is considered standard of care in the United States and has saved countless lives and limbs.

You can take this simple routine and expand it to have meaning in your own life because what you do and the path you choose to take represent high stakes.

Verifying the patient's name is like stopping to reflect on who you are as an individual. During this time-out, you can verify your personal values and your professional goals.

The next step is to verify the procedure. This is like asking, what is my career? What is my life's pathway? What do I really want to do? In other words, do you see an alignment with the path you are currently on and the vision you have for yourself?

The next is to verify your location. Ask yourself if you want to do a job in a particular setting, such as close to friends and family, in a big city, or in the country. Just as in real estate, "location, location, location" can be critical.

Lastly, we always check the consent form before we begin a procedure, and this is like a mental check to give yourself permission to make any personal or professional changes to avoid or reverse burnout. Keeping an open mind, ask if it's time to change your work, change your outlook, or change your goals.

MAKE A PERSONAL CHECKLIST

Taking a time-out goes hand-in-hand with having a personal checklist, which you should consult before making your next move. The idea goes back to the pre-flight checklists that every pilot does before takeoff. Perhaps surprisingly, this precautionary exercise had not initially been a standard feature of aircraft operation.

According to researcher and writer Atul Gawande, in 1935, the prototype Boeing B-17 Flying Fortress bomber (then known as the Model 299) crashed shortly after takeoff from Wright Field in Dayton, Ohio, killing both pilots. An investigation found that prior to take-off, the pilots had forgotten to disengage the crucial "gust locks," devices that stop control surfaces from moving in the wind while parked. With the control surfaces locked, it was impossible to fly the airplane properly. Aviation critics declared the advanced four-engine plane was "too advanced to fly," meaning that its various systems and controls were too complex for a human pilot to manage.

The Army Air Corps was ready to cancel the contract, but in

response, engineers at the Boeing Company developed a pre-flight checklist to ensure that pilots did not rely on their memories when preparing for takeoff. It required the pilot to recite a list of actions that had to be taken before takeoff, and the co-pilot checked each item to verify it was correct. It worked, and pilots were able to fly the B-17 safely. Soon after this system was implemented in the military, it was adopted by commercial airlines, ultimately becoming a practice within aviation throughout the world.[55]

Do you have a personal checklist? Your work/life synergy proceeds through years, months, weeks, days, hours, and even minutes. Life can get complicated, and with a checklist, you can stay organized, keep your priorities in order, and avoid distractions.

You may do this on a daily basis with a personal checklist of things you want to accomplish in one day. Such lists can be pretty simple, such as the grocery list you take to the supermarket. This particular list is important to curtail impulse buying. You may also have a daily calendar of appointments. If you're self-employed, this list might be short, but if you're the CEO of a big or fast-growing company, your daily calendar might be very detailed and planned to the minute, with little flexibility.

No matter what form your list takes, it functions the same way as a pre-flight checklist: It relieves you of the burden of having to remember everything you need to do and prevents you from forgetting important tasks or appointments. It also gives you the opportunity to pause and review where you are in your day.

You may also have a broader checklist of goals you want to reach in the next year, five years, or 10 years. This may include such things as buying a home, getting a degree or certification, reaching a certain income, paying off a debt, or being promoted to a particular position. If you have big goals, you'll want to break them down into smaller steps.

For example, if one of your goals is to earn a degree, you'll need to find a program, determine the financial requirements, apply for loans and grants, ensure your regular work is not impacted (or if it is, make the necessary arrangements), take any required tests, and submit your application.

Periodically, you can take some time to review your list to gauge your progress. How does all of this affect your ability to work happy and avoid burnout? It puts you in control of your daily activities and prevents you from dropping the ball on projects or plans you want to do. Remember, job burnout isn't only about the boredom from doing a repetitive job or putting up with difficult conditions; it's also about the deep fatigue you feel when you're constantly dealing with unexpected challenges that you could have planned for.

Ask yourself: Do you have a checklist of what you want to accomplish today and in the long term? Are you ready to move forward, or do you need more preparation? Are there any roadblocks ahead or have they been cleared? Putting your work on hold for just a few minutes to answer these questions can help you to work happy and avoid needless mistakes that, if they become cumulative, can lead to burnout.

CHAPTER 8

Self-Help Strategies: Make Small Changes

THE THEME OF THIS BOOK is that "work" and "life" are not distinct universes. You are the same person at home as you are at work. You don't leave home with one personality and arrive at work with another. The best way to work happily and avoid burnout is to do what you love, pace yourself, and be able to look back on what you've accomplished with pride.

For example, let's say Joe and Fred each work as executive chefs in a big hospital. Their job is to supervise the making and serving of a variety of foods for the hospital workers and guests who patronize the cafeteria and for the patients who have food sent to their rooms. One of the menu choices is pizza. The pizza is of good quality; they're not just slapping cheese and tomato sauce on a frozen crust.

Joe and Fred approach their jobs with two very different attitudes.

1. Joe, who works at City Hospital, tells himself he's in it for the paycheck and doesn't really care about pizza. It's just not his thing. He tells his staff to keep expenses down and not worry about the patients. "Where else are they going to eat?" he asks. "We have a captive audience." When he goes home at night, he's ready to forget his job because it's just a way to pay the bills.

2. Fred, who works at Lake General Hospital, has a different attitude. He's dedicated to making the very best pizza in any hospital. He's interested in the ingredients and their quality. He asks his chef to experiment with new combinations of toppings. He eats the pizza himself and even distributes comment cards in the cafeteria, soliciting feedback from his customers. His goal is to ensure a positive dining experience at Lake General Hospital.

Here's the question: Who will be working happy, Joe or Fred?

If they both stay with their jobs, Fred will be working happy and avoiding burnout. Even though Joe and Fred are doing the same thing, Fred loves his work, while to Joe, it's just a boring paycheck job. Fred sees the big picture; his goal is to make his customers happy, and making pizza just happens to be the skill he possesses and can use.

This leads to an important question: Is Joe a bad guy? Should we condemn him?

No. Joe is not a bad guy. He's just in the wrong line of work. He's not interested in pizza or making his customers happy. His interests lie elsewhere. So, what should Joe do? Ideally, Joe should find work that matches his life or change his perspective and learn to find joy in what he does. We don't know what that is, but Joe owes it to himself to find out.

Work and life should be inseparable. It's not necessarily a question of the allocation of time; it's about how we choose to think and use our energy. We must realize that life is much more than the fact that we're simply breathing. Life is more than existence; it's that you are conscious of yourself and your surroundings. When you recognize that you are life, you become more careful with how you choose to use it.

FREE YOURSELF FROM DISTRACTIONS

One of the most effective things you can do at work to stay happy and avoid burnout is to prioritize what you do and not get bogged down with tasks that don't really matter.

We're not talking about overwork due to circumstances beyond your control. Thousands of nurses and doctors at the height of the COVID-19 pandemic were physically and mentally overwhelmed by the huge surge of patients needing critical care. They were simply forced to do more than they could handle.

I'm talking about a normal workday where the time seems to slip away, and suddenly you find yourself scrambling to finish before 5:00 p.m. There are several causes of this type of time-wasting; here are the biggies.

Procrastination. It's a natural human tendency to put off chores that are painful or challenging. Instead, we divert our attention to little things that we tell ourselves are important. We say we need to fiddle with a spreadsheet, review a report, clean our desk, take a walk to the other end of the building — anything to avoid tackling a difficult job.

The cure for procrastination is to *embrace the challenge.* Solving a big problem is much more satisfying than skirting the edges, but only if you love what you do. The reason you procrastinate is because your heart just isn't in your work. Try to discover something about your work that you love, or find tasks that excite you. Then you'll be less likely to procrastinate.

Putting out fires. This syndrome can be a major source of burnout. Do you find yourself responding to every call for help from a manager or colleague? The phone rings or someone comes to your office with a problem, and you want to help, so you drop what you're doing and rush to their aid. Even if you fix the problem, you may be hurting yourself and the company because you've ignored or deferred one of your own responsibilities, which you now have to scramble to address.

This problem is indicative of a lack of planning within a culture of chaos. As an employee who must respond to sudden and often avoidable situations, you can help yourself by asking your manager for clarity on any issue or task that may have problems. For example, if a shipment of parts is scheduled to arrive, you could ask your boss if there's a contingency plan in case the parts are late or defective. With contingency plans in place, if the need arises, you can quickly pivot and not waste time.

Busy work. Busy work is where you trick yourself into thinking you're being productive, but in reality, you're performing meaningless tasks that don't get you any closer to completing your goals. A favorite piece of busy work is checking your email every few minutes. Usually, this is pointless and results in no new information, but it's a surprisingly powerful habit that, for significant psychological reasons, many people find hard to break. Experts say don't go "cold turkey," but try slightly lengthening the time between checking. For instance, if you currently check it every 30 minutes, try every 40 minutes. Then, stretch that to once per hour.

Be clear on what you need to accomplish. Dedicate yourself to focusing on one key task at a time. And don't worry about your boss — if she needed to get hold of you right away, she'd call you on the phone.

Distraction. When you're working out of direct sight of your supervisor, whether from your office cubicle or a warehouse or a job in the field, it's easy to become distracted by things around you. Today, your phone and its various apps are major culprits of distracted work. Instagram, TikTok, X (formerly Twitter), YouTube, Candy Crush Saga — they're all right there on your phone, vying for your attention.

A 2020 survey by Screen Education revealed that employees waste, on average, 2.5 hours per day "accessing digital content that is unrelated to their job." In an office, this is a waste of time, while in an industrial setting, it can be dangerous: Among respondents who worked in industry, a whopping 26% reported accidents had occurred in their workplace because someone was distracted by their smartphone.[56]

How can being distracted by your phone and its apps burn you out? Isn't it possible that by "taking a break" to play Call of Duty, you'll stay interested in your job?

No. It doesn't work that way. When you find yourself playing games or watching cat videos on TikTok during work hours, it means two things:

1. You're disengaged from your job, which is not a good thing and produces burnout.
2. You're filling your brain full of nonsense and gibberish, which actually could become addictive.

In fact, smartphones being habit-forming led to their inclusion in the 5th edition of the *Diagnostic and Statistical Manual of Mental Disorders*, the psychiatric diagnostic bible. Cell phone addiction manifests in various ways, including loss of interest in activities, anxiety when you cannot send or receive messages, and irritability when you're away from your phone. At work or at school, too much smartphone usage decreases the attention span and, according to numerous studies, contributes to increased rates of depression.[57]

EXERCISE YOUR RIGHT TO DISCONNECT

When you're at home in the evening, are you available for messages from work? When you wake up in the morning, do you immediately grab your phone to check your office emails or texts?

If so, your body may be at home, but your brain is still on the payroll. This is not a good idea; you should be willing and able to disconnect from your job. Too often, we stay glued to the phone and become addicted to work instead of enjoying what's in front of us, such as our partner, kids, or nature.

Take the time you need to prepare and refresh your mind.

In fact, some countries have passed laws prohibiting after-work contact from an employer. France, noted for its 35-hour work-week, pioneered such a law when, in 2017, it granted workers the right to ignore work communications outside of working hours.

"Employees physically leave the office, but they do not leave their work. They remain attached by a kind of electronic leash — like a dog," Parliamentarian Benoit Hamon told the BBC at the time.[58]

Italy, Belgium, Spain, Ireland, and Portugal have adopted similar laws, giving employees the "right to disconnect," as it's called.

Unfortunately, on a national basis, the United States has been slow to embrace the idea. Maybe it's because of our ingrained sense of competition or because it's rooted in our culture. Maybe it's because we don't know any better, or it's how we have always done it. But think about this: Before the age of digital communications (that is to say, way back in the year 2000), when you went home from work, your boss, colleague, or client had *no way to contact you* except by calling you on your landline phone, which they would never do except in the most dire emergency. It was taken for granted that when you left the office at the end of the day, you were *gone* until the next morning, and what you did in the meantime was nobody's business.

And yet, somehow, despite being out of reach of the office, we got our work done.

The importance of disconnecting applies not just to work but to social media at home. We need to practice energy preservation throughout the day, but especially in the evening. This means limiting our engagement with social media and, at times, even the news.

The solution? Set aside one hour every day just for yourself, and tell everyone that your day has only 23 hours in it. During that one hour (this is the minimum — it could be longer!), put your phone in the drawer. Use that hour to rest your mind, center yourself, meditate, take a walk, sit outside, and chase a squirrel with your dog — whatever calms you and makes you realize that you are fully alive.

While being able to work happy at a career you love might mean making big changes, like switching jobs or even industries, it might also mean making many small changes. This is because over time, small annoyances and problems can build up and get bigger until you take action to correct them. Every day, take your own temperature, so to speak, and determine areas of friction and unhappiness; then take the necessary steps to put yourself into alignment with what you truly want.

BE KIND TO YOURSELF

Many people can be harsh on themselves and then ask, "Why am I not happy?"

Think about this: If you don't get along with yourself, then how can you like anyone else? Begin by being kind to yourself, forgiving to yourself, and loving to yourself. When was the last time you complimented yourself? Instead of looking in the mirror and complaining about your wrinkles, try saying, "Good morning, Good Looking!" Even if it makes you chuckle, the positive energy created means it was a successful experiment — not in an arrogant way, but just appreciative of yourself.

Are you your own worst enemy? Don't focus on what is *wrong* with you; focus on what is *right* with you. Someone might say, "I need to control my temper, and then I will be a better person." This is success with strings attached. You're putting a qualification in front of your happiness and work/life synergy. You're saying, "I cannot be happy until, and unless, I change a particular personality defect," "until I acquire a particular skill," or "until my circumstances change."

Forget the qualifications. Love yourself and be happy *now*. If you hate your job, envision a better future state where you love your job and take action to make that dream a reality.

You need to accept who you truly are and acknowledge that you're in the process of changing. Everyone has struggles. We're not intended to ever be a "finished" product, static and unchanging. You need to accept who you are while life molds you. Any mistake you have made in your life is just that: a mistake. It doesn't change your fundamental purpose in life. Don't magnify your failures. There will always be areas to improve on.

Someone else might say, "I want that promotion or raise, and then I will be happy." Well, you may not be where you want to be, but at least you're not where you once were. Think about how far you have already come, not how far you have to go. It's how you train yourself to think. Do you focus on the times you won or the times you lost? Realize there is not one other person on this planet like you. You are special, and no one can be you better than you. Don't try to be like someone else.

NO MORE WORKCATIONS, WOLIDAYS, BLEISURE TRAVEL...

In recent years, and particularly after the COVID-19 pandemic, the idea of a "workcation," "woliday," or "bleisure" (business-leisure travel) has metastasized. This is basically the ability of remote workers to do their jobs from far-flung locales by logging into the office from, say, a resort in the Bahamas or a ski lodge in the Rocky Mountains.

This has long been the aspiration of freelancers and so-called digital nomads, and it is becoming a reality for millions of desk jockeys. The travel industry is promoting the trend; a recent report by Deloitte says that "laptop-lugging leisure travelers" took to the skies twice as often during the end of 2022 as traditional vacationers.[59]

But as writer Gloria Liu noted, we all need to regularly take a clean and complete break from our work,[60] and this happens via six mechanisms:

1. Detachment, when we mentally disengage from work.
2. Relaxation, which means doing pleasant activities that demand very little effort.
3. Autonomy, by which we dictate our own schedules.
4. Mastery of experiences that deliver a sense of competence outside of work.
5. Meaning as a sense of a purpose in what we do outside of work.
6. Affiliation, which means making a connection with others outside of work.

A good vacation and break from work should offer all six elements, represented by the acronym DRAMMA.

If you take your show on the road, so to speak, and combine work with watching the sunset from your hotel balcony in Maui, you're getting a change of scenery, but you're definitely *not* benefitting from the full effects of DRAMMA:

1. Detachment — No. You're still tied to the office.
2. Relaxation — Somewhat. You have more free time because you're not commuting.
3. Autonomy — No. You're still tied to the office on the usual schedule.
4. Mastery of experiences — Maybe, because it's easy to close your laptop and jump into the ocean.
5. Meaning — Nope. Not much opportunity for that.
6. Affiliation — Possibly. You'll get to know the hotel bartender pretty well.

While a workcation or woliday might be an interesting diversion once, it's no substitute for getting work out of your brain for an extended length of time. Again, consider the words of Leonardo da Vinci: "Every now and then go away, have a little relaxation, for when you come back to your work your judgment will be surer."

He meant *go away*. He did not mean answer messages from Rome or deal with wealthy clients demanding paintings.

A German research study found that healthy psychological detachment from work during leisure time means that the employee mentally disconnects from work and does not think about job-related issues when they're off the job. The employee who experiences true detachment from work during off-hours is *more satisfied* with their life and experiences fewer symptoms of psychological strain without being less engaged while at work.[61]

And here's the real problem: Many employees think workcations are just another way for employers to avoid providing real paid time off (PTO). According to a report by the Center for Economic and Policy Research, the United States is the only advanced economy in the world that does not guarantee its workers any paid vacation time. As a result, 25% of private-sector workers in the U.S. do not receive *any* paid vacation or paid holidays.

The report "No-Vacation Nation" revealed that European workers are guaranteed at least 20 paid vacation days per year, with as much as 30 days in some countries. Even in workaholic Japan, employees are guaranteed 10 paid days off per year. The sweetest deals are in Portugal and Austria, both of which provide a total of 35 paid vacation and holidays per year.[62]

These are numbers that American workers can only dream of.

The sneaky kind of workcation is one that interrupts or replaces your vacation. It might look like a vacation, but doesn't involve disconnecting or unplugging from your job. Our smartphones and laptops make it too easy. We're connected 24/7. When work emails come through to the device that never leaves your side, they're impossible to ignore.

Think about vacations in the 20th century: You went to your cabin in the woods, and the only link you had to the outside world was the rotary phone in the kitchen, which was connected to a landline. The people in your office might not have the number; you could call them (if you wanted), but they couldn't call you.

Today, you may be sitting on a beach in Jamaica, but you're neither fully at work nor fully at play. Instead, you're in a kind of purgatory, the worst of both worlds. It's work in vacation's clothing. It's not a legitimate employee benefit.

Here's another activity that contributes to burnout: eating lunch at your desk like a slave on a Roman galley chained to his oar. A study from EZcater, an online marketplace that connects businesses and catering companies, revealed that one in 10 employees don't take breaks away from their desk, and 70% of employees work through lunch at least once a week.

Executives are not immune: At least three times per week, 56% of director-level and 51% of vice presidents (and above) work at their desks while eating lunch.

Not only are those workers — dubbed "desktop diners" in the report — losing precious breaks to email and Zoom meetings, they may actually be less productive. The report found that "stopping to eat and taking mental breaks can prevent burnout — especially in the context of the extra stressful times workers have faced over the past few years."[63]

MANAGE EXPECTATIONS

While it's impossible to make your expectations of some future event match the reality of that event when it happens, to work happy and avoid burnout in your career, you must be able to get them pretty close.

We've all heard stories about friends or family members, or have experienced ourselves, the scenario where you accept a new job with great excitement and anticipation, only to be crushed when the reality of the job hits home. Maybe the boss who was super-sweet in the onboarding process turns out to be a jerk, or the job is boring, or the management is clueless. Whatever the reason, what should have been a dream role turns out to be a nightmare.

Employers take measures to protect themselves from unpleasant surprises when they hire. You've probably heard the expression, "Hire slow, fire fast." Employers interpret this to mean that they should take their time to ensure a new employee is a good fit before making a permanent hire, and conversely, if an employee turns out to be a bad fit, they should be dismissed promptly.

As an employee, your expression should be "Join slow, assimilate fast." Taking your time can be a challenge because many employees need the income and will grab the first good-paying job offer they receive. Try not to do this. Try to spend as much time as possible with your prospective employer before saying "yes."

At the end of the day, true deep happiness, what the ancient Greeks called *eudaimonia*, or behavior of the soul in accord with virtue, comes from within you. Do yourself a favor and have reasonable expectations of your job, coworkers, and rewards. There is no perfect job. Don't try to find something that does not exist.

KEEP IT REAL

A few years ago, comedian Adam Sandler did a skit on *Saturday Night Live* that captured this reality perfectly. He played a tour operator who took groups of American tourists to the historic cultural sites of Italy. In his pitch for Romano Tours, Sandler made it clear to his customers that if they were miserable on Long Island, they'd still be miserable in Florence. A trip to Italy had no power to lift them from their depression.

"If you're sad now," he said, "you might still feel sad there. If you're sad where you are, and then you get on a plane to Italy, you in Italy will be the same sad you were before, just in a new place." He added that a trip to Italy "cannot fix deeper issues, like how you behave in group settings or your general baseline mood. That's a job for incremental lifestyle changes sustained over time. This may sound rude, but I'm trying to temper expectations."[64]

Just as a trip to Italy with Romano Tours will not solve your personal issues, landing your "dream job" but *not having any other life* is a recipe for disaster.

At first, this may seem like a contradiction, because this book is all about finding deep fulfillment in the work you do to pay your bills. That's still true and always will be true; however, this book is also about work/life synergy, and if you're not happy *outside* of your dream job, your life will eventually become a nightmare despite your job initially satisfying all of the boxes on your checklist.

No matter how wonderful your job is, you need to step away from it on a regular basis. You need to go home every day for a break, every weekend for a longer break, and at least two weeks every year for an even longer break. While you're not at work, you shouldn't just sit and stare at the walls or watch TV; you need to engage your brain in some activity that uses different skills than your job requires.

Warren Buffett invests all day reading financial reports and then goes home and plays bridge or practices his ukulele. He disengages his brain from his work, which keeps him happy and helps him avoid burnout.

Ask yourself: What do you do outside of work to recharge? Do you feel you can entirely disconnect from work when you go home or on vacation? I hope you can.

THE POWER OF GRATITUDE

The word "gratitude" is derived from the Latin *gratia,* which means "grace," "graciousness," or "gratefulness." It's a thankful appreciation for what we receive, whether tangible or intangible. By expressing gratitude, we acknowledge the goodness in our lives while recognizing that the source of that goodness lies, at least partially, outside ourselves. As a result, being grateful also helps us connect to something larger than ourselves as individuals, whether it's to nature, other people, or a higher power.

In positive psychology research, gratitude is strongly and consistently associated with greater personal happiness. It helps us feel more positive emotions, improve our health, cherish good experiences, build strong relationships, and deal with adversity.

The opposite of feeling gratitude is feeling aggrieved or victimized and dwelling on those feelings. Research has shown that attitude can affect health. In one study, two psychologists, Robert A. Emmons of the University of California-Davis, and Michael E. McCullough of the University of Miami, asked volunteers to write a few sentences each week focusing on particular topics. As reported by Harvard Health, one group wrote about things they were grateful for that had occurred during the week. Another group wrote about daily irritations or things that had displeased them. The third group wrote about events that had affected them, whether positive or negative.

After 10 weeks, the participants who wrote about gratitude were more optimistic and felt better about their lives. This same group also exercised more and had fewer visits to physicians than those who focused on sources of aggravation.[65]

It's all about where you place importance. If you make the good things in your life important, you'll be in alignment with them. If you make the unpleasant or negative things in your life important, you'll be in alignment with those.

If you're going to fulfill your destiny, instead of going around pitying yourself because you did something wrong or because something wasn't fair, change your perspective to an attitude of gratefulness for what you do have, an understanding that scars (physical or non-physical) don't disqualify you but actually prepare you for your future. A recognition that we all have something unique we can contribute to this world can fuel your passion and literally change the world.

Here's a personal story. My son just got into puzzles. The first time we did a puzzle together, we chose a puzzle box with a picture of a cool car that would be the end result of assembling its contents. He got all excited when he saw the car and couldn't wait for me to open the box. As I opened the box and dumped the pieces on the floor, I could see the disappointment in his eyes. . He picked up one of the oddly shaped pieces and said, "This is not a car!"

Isn't that the way life is sometimes? We're all made up of little pieces, which in isolation may not make any sense. They may look odd and not even very attractive, but when we put all those pieces together over the course of a lifetime, they come together, and even that oddly shaped piece has the perfect place in the beautiful picture we see on the outside of the box.

Be grateful for the little pieces of your life, the unique attributes you have, and the experiences you have. If it doesn't make sense now, it will in the future.

BETTER INPUTS = BETTER OUTPUTS

Your inputs influence your outputs. As they say in the computer business, "Garbage in, garbage out." I prefer to state it in a more positive way: "Good things in, good things out." What you watch, listen to, read, surround yourself with, say, and think about will be what you become. You need to monitor all of these inputs to your brain because they contribute to your output.

What do I watch? Well, my son is currently into *PJ Masks*. For those of you who aren't familiar with it, *PJ Masks* is a computer-animated superhero children's television series based on the *Les Pyjamasques* book series by Romuald Racioppo. When night falls, the human kids, Amaya, Greg, and Connor, become the superhero team PJ Masks in order to fight various enemies. Amaya becomes Owlette (an owl), Greg becomes Gekko (a lizard), and Connor becomes Catboy (a combination of cat and boy).

Like many kids, my son walks around the house pretending that he's Gekko while flexing his Super Gekko Muscles and later Super Gekko Camouflaging when it's bath time!

This is interesting because if I had no child, I would *never* watch *PJ Masks*. Being a rational grown-up, I have zero interest in the subject, yet I do watch it, and it's a window into a child's world (at least as envisioned by the Disney Jr. channel). In that sense, I'm grateful for the opportunity to see the world in the strange and fantastical way that children do. At a young age, they literally cannot tell the difference between fantasy and reality.

My son, and most kids his age, will insist that some crazy thing like a mermaid or a dragon is absolutely 100% real, and you're wasting your breath telling them otherwise. But this is a wonderful thing and — this is true — it's a great antidote to grown-up burnout and cynicism. Why not believe in mermaids and dragons, at least a little bit?

In fact, the power of human imagination can lead to great things. Take, for example, mermaids, those human-like creatures who can swim underwater for long periods of time. For thousands of years, earthbound humans have imagined having the same powers, and people tried all sorts of devices to allow them to breathe underwater. The technology developed slowly, and in the 20th century came the big breakthrough.

In 1939, U.S. Army Major Christian J. Lambertsen invented an underwater free-swimming oxygen rebreather, and in 1952 he patented a modification of his apparatus, which he named SCUBA, an acronym for "self-contained underwater breathing apparatus." Then, the famous undersea explorer Jacques Cousteau co-invented an improved device he called the Aqua-Lung, allowing divers to remain submerged for a much longer time and go deeper than ever before. Suddenly, swimming underwater like a mythical mermaid was something that nearly anyone could do — all because humans imagined having that power and worked to make it a reality.

Here's an interesting thing about Jacques Cousteau, who was born in 1910. In 1933, he became an officer in the French Navy, where his interest lay not in diving but in aviation. He wanted to be a navy pilot. Unfortunately, he was in a serious automobile accident in which both of his arms were broken. The injury affected his ability to fly an aircraft and led to his disqualification from the aviation program. Instead of bemoaning his terrible fate, he turned to his second love: the sea. The rest, as they say, is history, and through his films and TV shows, Jacques Cousteau became synonymous with undersea exploration.

THE COMPANY YOU KEEP

If you look at anyone who's successful and happy in their work, you'll find they surround themselves with like-minded people who share their positive attitude. As a group, they have a common goal and see themselves as sharing responsibilities and rewards. While each person may be a specialist in his or her area, there's a spirit of collaboration. It's captured by the old English expression, "Many hands make light work" — at least as long as all the hands are united by a common vision.

Just as you bring your attitude to a collaborative effort and influence others with it, the attitudes of your teammates can rub off on you. This can be either positive or negative.

On the negative side, if your workplace colleagues are incessantly complaining about their jobs, eventually they can erode your own perception of a job you may actually like.

Insincere behavior can be corrosive as well. We can think of certain public figures who are known to surround themselves with "yes-men" who don't challenge them and tell them what they want to hear. Such people are deeply insecure and, because they live in an echo chamber, often make poor decisions.

The people with whom you spend the most time have a big influence on how you view the world, your moods, and the expectations you have of yourself. When you surround yourself with others who are working happy, you're more likely to adopt empowering beliefs and see life as happening *for* you instead of *to* you. In a sense, this is a healthy manifestation of the law of attraction. This is a belief that your mind can shape your destiny, and if you *believe* good things will happen for you, they will. But if you believe bad things will happen to you, they will.

There's truth to this in terms of how you approach success and failure. It's not literally true for every event in life, however. For example, you obviously have no control over whether a tornado is going to hit your neighborhood. Your personal belief in tornadoes is not relevant; if it comes, it comes. But you have tremendous control over *how you prepare to survive a tornado*, such as with the proper insurance and a secure, stormproof cellar in your house. You have power over *how you recover from a tornado*.

This is the real power of attraction. The same applies to your job. If you have a winning attitude and your co-workers have the same attitude, your success will be greater, and your setbacks will be less costly. You'll be working happy and with no burnout.

It takes a certain kind of humility to seek out the company of people who not only share your positive vision but who are more advanced than you in their education or experience; however, the smarter you are, the more likely you are to do just that. Jack Ma, the Chinese business magnate, investor, philanthropist, and co-founder and former executive chairman of Alibaba Group, said, "I hire someone smarter than me, and I think, 'In four or five years, he can be my boss. I would like to work for him.'"

Making these decisions takes both humility and self-confidence. Someone with that humble attitude is focused on success and isn't concerned about ego. They look forward to going to work every day because they know they're going to learn something new from the people around them.

THE POWER OF WORDS

What we think about and what we say are critically important. Words have incredible power. When you *speak* it, even whisper it to yourself, you can become what you say. Your life moves in the direction of your words.

You have to say it before you will see it.

You can't talk defeat and expect victory.

You can't be negative and expect to live a positive life.

A poor mouth equals a poor life.

If you want to succeed, you have to be your own cheerleader. You can't let other people's negative voices about you or your workplace drown out your own internal positive thoughts.

Go ahead — dare to declare it! Words are like seeds that we plant in the ground. Once spoken, they begin to take root within us, and over time, we will become what we are saying.

Don't use words to *describe* a situation; use words to *change* the situation. Especially during difficult times, it's easy to talk about the problem, but talking about it makes it bigger than it needs to be. Stop talking about the problem and start talking about the plan. Instead of "I didn't get the promotion," say, "One door closes, and another will open." In other words, don't talk *about* the problem; talk *to* the problem. "I see what the situation is, and this is what I'm going to do about it."

This approach is related to neuro-linguistic programming, a self-improvement system introduced by Richard Bandler and John Grinder in their 1975 book *The Structure of Magic I*. The idea is that you can re-wire your brain and get it on a positive track by speaking affirmatively, out loud, and with other behavioral techniques. It's a complicated methodology, but the gist of it is that by *modeling* what you aspire to be, you can *become* what you want to be. If you want to become a leader, then start talking and acting like one. Obviously, you can't just march around and give people orders; what we're talking about is a state of mind and an attitude. Set your sights on a future desired state and behave as if you're already there.[66]

Many people have diarrhea of the mind; they are trapped in the drama they create and not in the world they're living in. If you go to the gym, pick up a five-pound weight, and do bicep curls, no matter how strong you are, if you do them long enough, your arm will hurt. If you never stop flexing your bicep, even a small weight can cause pain and eventual discomfort. The same is true with your mind. If thoughts keep coming and coming and coming, no matter how strong you are, if you don't take a break, you eventually will get a headache and feel burned out.

How do you address this? When you have diarrhea of the gut, we all know things can get bad quickly. The first thing you do is stop eating. Generally, this is followed by rest and a few trips to the toilet.

When you have diarrhea of the mind, you are unable to control your mind, your thoughts, and your emotions, and what you say will reflect this shortcoming. You say things that hurt others, and your mind gravitates to the negative. The treatment for this negativity consists of these six steps:

1. **Stop talking.** As the slang expression goes, "Zip it!" Not every thought you have in your mind needs to take shape in your mouth. For the moment, restrict your speaking only to communications that are absolutely necessary. Appreciate the value of each word you utter.

2. **Listen.** People who are insecure often confuse *listening* with *acceptance*. They are two very different things. You can listen to another person and understand what they say without agreeing with them or abandoning your own beliefs. Listening is not a sign of weakness; it's actually a sign of strength. If you say to someone who seems to be adversarial, "I will listen to what you have to

say," your act can calm them down and make them less afraid and therefore, more comfortable listening to you.

Be patient as you listen. Let the other person finish. Inspirational author/speaker Simon Sinek advises, "There is a difference between listening and waiting for your turn to speak."

3. **Take a rest.** Let the waters grow still and the dust settle. Consider your own thoughts. Do they make sense? What is their intention: to heal or to injure? To make yourself look enviable in the eyes of others or to elevate others? Think about what's most important to you. Do you really need to win an argument or insist that your point of view prevail?

4. **Ask yourself why you feel the way you do.** Each of us develops a point of view based on our own experiences, often going back to when we were children. We all have biases, many of which are harmless but some of which can be destructive. The destructive biases can make agreements impossible and can distort our perspective. It takes maturity and wisdom to look in the mirror and tell yourself that you understand and accept the reality of your own biases, and pledge to try to minimize their impact on how you relate to other people.

5. **Have empathy.** Just as you should ask yourself why you feel the way you do, it's just as important to ask yourself why the other person might feel the way they do. Consider your thoughts from an opposing viewpoint. Since no two people on the planet are the same, it's more than likely that your perspective will differ from that of other persons.

To illustrate, let's say your manager is in a foul mood and snaps at you for what you consider a minor error. Your first emotional response might be to think, "What a jerk! That's the last time I'm ever going to make an extra effort for him — or for this lousy company!" Instead, you take a deep breath and center yourself and recognize this truth: When another human being lashes out at you, they are doing nothing other than *revealing their own inner pain.*

Think of reasons why your manager might be uptight. Is he under pressure from his boss? Remember, every person who draws a paycheck has a boss — even the CEO, who must answer to the board and the shareholders. Does she have a personal issue at home? Even though employees are supposed to leave their personal problems at the door, we're all human, and it can be difficult to keep your mind off some issue outside of work. Does he have a deadline or task that he's worried about? Has she gotten a bad report?

Then think about this: Aside from your wounded pride, have you suffered any injury? This is not to say that anyone should be expected to accept poor treatment, but people who succeed in this world are able to step back, see a situation objectively, and not take offense when someone reveals their personal pain.

6. **Offer positivity.** When you speak, it's easy to point out all the imperfect, thoughtless, and damaged things in the world. Identifying a problem is the first step toward solving it. To point to it without offering a solution is, in many ways, worse than saying nothing. Use your voice as an instrument to bring positive change to the world. Offer encouragement and praise and stay focused on the future.

This section of the book has revealed how you can make changes within yourself to keep working happy and avoid becoming burned out. Your inner changes should always be for the betterment of you, your family, and your community. As human beings, we're actually much more flexible and adaptive than we give ourselves credit for, which is a good thing. In the next chapter, we're going to dig deeper to discover what may never change inside of you: your purpose.

CHAPTER 9

Your Purpose in
Work and Life

IN THE FIRST EIGHT CHAPTERS of this book, we've explored the choices you can make as you aspire to achieve work/life synergy — that is to say, the ultimate combination of career and home life that keeps you excited and energized about both. Many of these strategies focus on how you can change from within to successfully manage and even grow to love the realities of life in the working world. You might call it the approach of "When life gives you lemons, make lemonade."

Or even better yet, "When life gives you lemons, plant them, grow a lemon tree orchard, and enjoy a prosperous life."

It's not about "selling out" or willfully becoming a cog in the great machine; it's all about finding dignity and satisfaction in the work you do, regardless of its degree of difficulty.

We've explored the possibilities of changing your job and even your career so that you'll be more aligned with how you envision your life and closer to your ideal work/life synergy.

The beginning and the end of this process should be the same: your "work" and your "life" happily intertwined and working in synergy with each other, with the interaction of the two producing a positive effect greater than the sum of their separate effects.

This is a modern-day concern that our immediate ancestors didn't have. If you go back to the pre-industrial era, spanning thousands of years of human history up until the 19th century, there was no division between your work (meaning your occupation) and your life. They were inseparable. If you walked down the street in medieval London or Paris, you could identify the occupations of people by the clothes they wore. The butcher wore certain specified garb, as did the tailor, the clerk, the banker, the priest, the farmer, the herder. Even your surname reflected your occupation: Smith, Farmer, Baker,

Carpenter, Mason, Miller, Tanner, and many more. If you were John Weaver, everyone knew your occupation. You likely resided where you worked. If you were a barber, you probably lived above your shop.

Your access to formal education was extremely limited. Most ordinary people — farmers and tradespeople — were trained from childhood for an occupation typically chosen by the father. Apprenticeship was the common path. This meant that at age 10 or 12, you signed a contract with an established tradesperson. The contract stipulated that your benefactor would put you to work, teach you the trade (tanning, smithing, baking, whatever), and provide room and board for a certain number of years. When the contract was up, you qualified to join the guild of the trade for which you had been trained. And that was it — you were set up for life.

In more recent history, one of the most well-known apprentices was Benjamin Franklin. Born in 1706, he was one of 17 (yes, 17) children born to Josiah Franklin, a Puritan immigrant. Josiah wanted Benjamin to enter the clergy, but he could not afford his son's education. Because young Benjamin loved to read, Josiah decided that he should enter the printing and publishing business. At age 12 (the "age of reason"), Benjamin signed an indenture for his apprenticeship with his older brother, James Franklin, who owned a print shop in Boston. The contract obligated Benjamin until he turned 21, and only then would he be free to earn his own wages.

Young Benjamin embraced his position and undertook an ambitious program of self-development. He educated himself by reading the books he helped to print and taught himself persuasive writing by imitating the articles and opinion pieces. He also endured regular beatings from James because, in those days, corporal punishment was a common practice.

When Benjamin was 15, James founded *The New-England Courant*, one of the first American newspapers. But two years later, far short of his day of legal liberation, Benjamin reportedly had a violent dispute with James and fled as a fugitive to Philadelphia. While on the run, Benjamin secured jobs in printing houses, but he was dissatisfied with his prospects and went to London, where he worked as a printer until he returned to Philadelphia in 1726 at the age of 20.

Although Benjamin remained in the profession his father had chosen for him, he became a serial entrepreneur with wide-ranging interests. By 1748, at age 42, Benjamin became wealthy enough to retire from active business and live off his investments. He put away his leather apron, the traditional uniform of the printer, and became a gentleman, a legally recognized social position in the 18th century. He publicized his new station in life by having his portrait painted wearing a velvet coat and a brown wig. He also acquired a coat of arms and moved to a luxurious house in "a more quiet Part of the Town." And as a gentleman, he was free to pursue his true love: "Philosophical Studies and Amusements."[67]

The Industrial Revolution, which was just emerging in Franklin's later years, wiped out the old system. People began working in factories and living elsewhere. Workers wore nondescript clothing, and their names didn't identify their trades. A woman working a loom in a textile mill could be named Sally Gardener, or Alice Brewer, or anything else. The tools of the trade were owned by the employer, who paid workers in cash and sent them home at the end of the day.

In the era before World War II, most people lived in rural areas or in the center of a city. Rural areas were sparsely populated farmland, while cities were centers of manufacturing. In the post-war era, however, especially in America, the growth of "bedroom communities" in the suburbs put increased distance between work and home. The great cities lost population and became business centers, deserted at night and on weekends. Concepts like municipal zoning took root, and instead of walking from home to the field or factory as workers once did, they now drove or took a train from a well-defined residential neighborhood to an industrial or business district.

In the 21st century, and especially in the post-Covid era, we're seeing increased decentralization of work and a tremendous growth in remote white-collar work, with business employees working from home. Home can be anywhere, from an apartment on the top floor of a downtown skyscraper, to a cabin in the woods, to a boat in the Caribbean. The home itself is becoming the place where family wealth is generated, which is actually a throwback to the old ways before the era of factories.

Workers are also mobile in terms of their loyalty to their employer. It's hard to believe that in the 1950s and 1960s, a stated goal of IBM was employment "from the cradle to the grave." In those days, a resume with a history of "job-hopping," that is, changing jobs more frequently than once every five years, was red-flagged by employers. Unless there was a good explanation for the frequent job changes, the applicant would be considered disloyal or unreliable as an employee.

Today, an increasing number of workers work on a project basis. In 1995, just 10% of the American workforce provided their products or services on a contract, non-employee basis. By 2015, that number had jumped to 15.8%. Interestingly, Americans *want* to be self-employed. According to a Dartmouth University study on self-employment, volunteers were asked the simple question: "Suppose you were working and could choose between different kinds of jobs. Which would you prefer: being an employee or being self-employed?" In response, 70.8% said that they wanted to be self-employed.[68]

You can see where this is going. While workers still face employment challenges, many factors are making it easier to do the work they want to do, when they want, and even where they want. It's becoming easier to find or create work for yourself that allows you to achieve a healthy work/life synergy.

YOUR PURPOSE

This brings us to the big question:

If you could create your own work/life synergy from scratch, what would it be?

There are only two conditions to the challenge:

1. You have to work at a job to make money to support yourself. The option to live as a "gentleman" or "gentlewoman" like Benjamin Franklin and pursue only philosophical studies and amusements while lounging in your velvet coat and brown wig is off the table.

2. Your work/life synergy must be legal and ethical. For example, running a Ponzi scheme to defraud innocent people is not allowed.

To begin our exploration, let's go back to our human trait that makes us unique in the animal kingdom: the ability to be aware of our current state and to imagine an improved future state.

We can see our present house and imagine ourselves living in a mansion.

We can look up at the moon and imagine traveling there.

We can see people suffering and imagine an end to that suffering.

Or, as John Lennon wrote,

"Imagine no possessions

I wonder if you can

No need for greed or hunger

A brotherhood of man"[69]

A better future state is more than having a fat bank account. With some important exceptions, which we'll discuss in this chapter, it's well-known that pursuing a shallow goal such as "make more money than my neighbor" is not satisfying and quickly leads to burnout. Money is a tool and a means to an end, but it's not the end itself. Even if you are poor and you say to yourself, "I need to be a millionaire," that doesn't provide you with a road map to action and, therefore results. Money is the result of your work, not the work itself.

Here's a mental exercise that can help you. Imagine that you wake up on a ship. You don't know where you've been and you don't know where you're going. Then the ship arrives at a port city. It's a foreign place, but everyone speaks your language. You disembark from the ship and approach an official sitting at a desk.

"Welcome to Metropolis," he says. "Here, everyone has a job. All the jobs pay the same amount. What's your line of work?"

"My line of work?"

"Yes. What would you like to do that will benefit society and make you happy?"

"Well, I may need some training."

"No problem," says the official. "Anything can be arranged. The only question is, what will be satisfying for you?"

What would you say in such a situation? What occupation and source of income would you choose?

The interesting thing about this scenario is that you can't engineer an answer by working backwards from the outcome — that is, your paycheck. You can't say, "Well, I'll make more money if I choose to be a lawyer rather than a toymaker, so I'd better be a lawyer." In reality, this makes sense because if you're smart and you apply yourself, you can make a comfortable living doing just about anything.

The quintessential example of this is the remarkable story of Joe Ades. Born in England in 1934, he engaged in various sales-related occupations until he emigrated to New York City in 1993. It was there he launched his business: selling $5 vegetable peelers on the streets of Manhattan. He would rise at dawn, dress in a fashionable tailored suit and tie, and assemble his little cart with a day's supply of carrots and potatoes along with the peelers that he bought wholesale. Then he'd march out of his Upper East Side apartment and, since he had no vendor's license, choose a different spot in park or on a street corner.

Sitting on a low stool so people were forced to approach him to see what he was doing, he'd launch into his captivating patter while demonstrating the peeler. He was part showman, part pitchman, and 100% confident in his ability to sell an ordinary vegetable peeler for $5. This was his daily routine until his death in 2009. His work enabled him to live comfortably on Park Avenue, enjoy café society at the Pierre Hotel, and send his children to college.

One day someone asked him if he ever took a vacation. He replied, "Life is a vacation! Every day is a vacation!"

As for his wealth, he said, "Never underestimate a small amount of money gathered by hand for 60 years."

And here's one more: When asked about the key to his success, he said, "Not doing what you like, but liking what you do. I think that's the secret of happiness."[70]

Let's go back to our hypothetical story about landing in a foreign city and having your choice of occupations. This is literally what happened to Joe Ades, and it happens to millions of immigrants every year. It also happens to high school and college graduates and to anyone who's been forced to start over in life, like Vera Wang when she failed to qualify for the Olympics. You stand there looking at your future, and you ask yourself three questions:

1. "What *can* I do? What skills do I have or can learn?"
2. "What do I *want* to do? What would give me pleasure? What would I do willingly?"
3. "What *should* I do? How can I best support my personal goals and those I care about?"

If you can find the intersection of these three questions and the answer they share in common, you will have found your purpose.

If you're still not sure about your skill set, look at it this way: What can you do to make *other people* happy? This takes the focus off you and turns the question around.

Can you make other people healthier?

Can you help them to be better informed?

Help them buy a house? Entertain them? Take them to see new places?

What could you do for other people that would give you a feeling of accomplishment and satisfaction?

This is the truest and most meaningful way to be working happy. The ancient Chinese advised, "If you want happiness for an hour, take a nap. If you want happiness for a day, go fishing. If you want happiness for a year, inherit a fortune. If you want happiness for a lifetime, help somebody."

And here's one from Abraham Lincoln: "To ease another's heartache is to forget one's own." This means that if you're focused on how you can help someone else lead a happier life, you'll be happier yourself.

Either way, you will achieve the work/life synergy you need to be working happy, knowing you're doing good for yourself and others.

A WORD ABOUT MONEY AS A MOTIVATOR

Every work/life book you read, including this one, will urge you to have a strong purpose to your work that's related to helping other people. Altruism is the most powerful motivating force we know, especially when the people we're helping are members of our own family.

With this advice generally comes the message that you shouldn't worry too much about the money, because if you find your true purpose and passion, the money will follow — *in that order*. Why is this true? Because money is nothing more than a medium of exchange. By itself, it has no value. You cannot eat a dollar bill. A billion bitcoin will not shelter you from the storm.

Money is simply a convenient way to avoid the headaches and inefficiencies of bartering. By using money, we can assign dollar values to all the things we need — bread, clothing, a car, a house — and we can also assign dollar values to our labor. With this simple symmetrical system, let's say you get paid $20 an hour for your labor, and a pair of jeans costs $20; now you know that if you work for an hour, you'll be able to buy a pair of jeans.

To earn money, you need to bring something of value to the marketplace. Whether this item of value is chickens or automobiles for sale, or your services as a doctor or business expert, it must be goods or services for which your customer is willing to exchange dollars.

This is why simply saying, "I'm going to make lots of money" or "I'm going to be a millionaire" is not practical; you are putting the result ahead of the process. You're chasing a reward that's disconnected from what you must do to *earn* that reward. The unavoidable questions become: "What *action* will you take in order to convince people to give you money? What *value* will you bring to the marketplace that you can then sell for money?"

That is true and will always be so, but it can be nuanced.

There are many situations in which a person can sincerely and truthfully turn the equation around by saying, "I will do *anything* to make more money. Making money is my single most important goal. Nothing else matters." Such a person is simply saying that he or she has an important goal to reach, and this goal requires money, and they're willing to do any job to earn it.

Here's an example. At the hospital where I work, I noticed that one of the maintenance men was always there, busy at his job. If I was there in the morning, Andre was busy cleaning. If I happened to be called in during the evening, I'd see Andre doing his job. It seemed like he never left! So finally, I asked him, "Say, Andre, don't you take any time off? You practically live here!"

He gave me a big smile and replied, "My wife and I have three children. We are determined that all three will go to college. It's a dream of ours. And we don't want them to have to be in debt. We want to pay for it. So, I work as many shifts as I can. If a shift opens up, I take it. The more money I can make, the more we have for their education."

Being a maintenance worker at a hospital is not an easy job. It's hard work, but Andre didn't care. His goal was to "bring home the bacon" for his family, with a specific goal: to raise enough cash to send his kids to college. For Andre, cash was king — but for a good reason.

Andre was also smart enough to know that the stream of cash flowing into his savings account depended upon his job performance. He did exceptional work, and he was always first choice of the facilities director when he had to fill a shift. For Andre, the formula was simple: Doing a good job at work no matter what = Having enough money to send kids to college = Deep personal pride and satisfaction.

Here's another example. For many people who have a large amount of debt, paying off that debt becomes their number one priority. That means generating as much cash income as possible while slashing their expenses. There are many stories of couples who paid off substantial student loan debt in just a year or two. One such story is about Ebony Horton and her husband, Justin, who were determined to pay off her $220,000 in undergraduate and grad school student loan debt. The Chicago-area couple were not wealthy people; as Ebony told *Business Insider*, "I was struggling to survive." She said she and Justin "had two cars, but I couldn't even afford to get a parking pass for the second car, so it was constantly getting towed. It was just one thing after another."[71]

With the help they received from her family with housing — the couple lived with her ailing grandparents for a year — they paid off the loans in three years. Horton and her husband put 95% of their combined incomes toward Horton's student loans, making payments of roughly $10,000 a month. It was not easy! She told *Forbes* magazine:

"We sacrificed our youth, our relationships…. We didn't travel, we missed out on family functions, and we worked seven days a week for almost a year.

"We chose to postpone having children. After my car broke down, I walked four miles to and from work…. We sacrificed our privacy, our sanity. It definitely put a strain on our marriage — we are still considered to be newlyweds; we've been married for three and a half years. But he was right by my side every step of the way and used his income to help pay off my loans."[72]

It sounds harrowing, but for Ebony and Justin, their relentless drive to maximize their income and minimize their expenses was to reach the goal of being free of debt. While they had some advantages — her parents gave her a condo they had purchased for $13,000 at a foreclosure auction, which she then rented out for more income — it's undeniable that they worked single-mindedly toward their goal. The last time their story appeared in the press, the couple was focused on buying rental properties to build a flow of passive income. Horton's mission, she said, was to retire at age 35.

Generally, someone who's relentlessly focused on making as much money as possible has one goal: to pay off debt and be free, to improve their life in some way, or to retire early in order to leave the 9-5 job market.

There's an exception to every rule, Warren Buffett! We've discussed his remarkable life, but two seemingly contradictory facts stand out:

1. His entire professional career is centered around making a profit from his investments. The only measure of his success is how much money he makes. The bigger the return on investment, the more successful he believes he's been.

2. He doesn't care about the money he makes. He buys no mansions or yachts. He lives in the same ordinary house he bought in 1958 for $31,500. Owning stuff doesn't interest him. He told the BBC, "How would I improve my life by having 10 houses around the globe? If I wanted to become a superin-

tendent of housing… I could have that as a profession, but I don't want to manage 10 houses, and I don't want somebody else doing it for me, and I don't know why the hell I'd be happier."[73] And he told CBS, "I have every possession I want. I have a lot of friends who have a lot more possessions. But in some cases, I feel the possessions possess them rather than the other way around."[74]

I think it's safe to say that Warren Buffett is, at heart, a person who likes to play games, and the game he chooses to play isn't chess or football or a TV quiz show, but investing. He plays that particular game better than anyone else.

OVERCOME YOUR FEAR OF THE FUTURE

Think about the number one thing that holds you back from leaping headfirst into your purpose. I mean this in a practical, day-to-day sense of getting up in the morning, going to work, seeing people, and interacting with them. And then you ask them to give you money for what you've done. This is the essence of it, isn't it? You can do whatever you want in life, but if what you do has no value to other people, no one's going to pay you, and you've got a problem. You could be a brilliant author of novels, but if no one buys them, you'll need to find some other way of earning money.

For many people, the fear of not having a steady and substantial income is their primary driving force. You can't blame them — it's no fun being poor. This is why they'll endure misery on the job. They don't see any alternative. The future is uncertain and even scary. The security of today's situation is preferable to the uncertainty of the future, especially if there's a major life change.

But people who aren't working happy have alternatives — two, in fact.

The first alternative is to find fulfillment in their current position. This does not mean accepting abuse. It means saying to yourself, "Okay, this is my reality. What can I find in this job that fulfills my purpose, allows me to use or further develop my skills, gives me pleasure, and makes me feel good about the contribution I'm making?

And how can I ignore or smooth over the parts that are difficult? What can I do outside of work to put my head into a good place to come back here every morning?"

It's good to remember that directly or indirectly, the goal of nearly every occupation is to improve the well-being of fellow humans, to solve some of their problems to make them happier or healthier, to provide food or shelter, or even to entertain them. This is the value you provide and for which you're compensated.

It's easier to see this in some fields than in others, but it's always there. Consider what should be an obvious example: my profession in healthcare. As a doctor, my purpose is to improve the health of my patients. I see patients, I treat them, and it's all about well-being. Every person who works in the healthcare industry, from the receptionist at the front desk to the most highly regarded brain surgeon, shares this same purpose.

You might think this worthwhile and valuable purpose would inoculate healthcare workers from job burnout. After all, we chose this profession, sacrificed decades of our life in training, and we can see its benefits in our patients. Yet reports say that over 50% of healthcare workers suffer from burnout.

Why is this?

I don't want to sound like I'm complaining, but the number one cause of healthcare worker burnout is all the stuff we must do that isn't directly related to caring for patients: the paperwork, phone calls, emails, demands from insurance payers, requirements for referral, lab tests, electronic medical record requirements, being judged on patient satisfaction, and more.

In 2021, doctors reported spending on average 15.6 hours per week on paperwork and other administrative tasks. This number has been rising steadily this century, even though the number of hours doctors spend *with their patients* has not changed. So where are these extra hours coming from? They're being added on to the end of the day. Longer hours, fewer breaks, more burnout.

What's the antidote to this? The only way to keep working happy is to understand and remember your purpose, which is to help people be healthier. By knowing and remembering their purpose, even the housekeepers in a hospital will realize they are not just cleaning a room, they are preventing dangerous infection. The receptionists know they are setting the tone for each patient's visit, ensuring the flow of patients is smooth and that every patient is treated with respect. The phlebotomists know they are properly collecting important blood samples to help diagnose the disease. The nurses know they are on the front lines of patient care, watching over their patients and providing lifesaving services. Every job can and should be done with pride. Every job should be respected because every job enhances human well-being in some capacity.

The second alternative is to take that leap into the unknown and find a new role that matches your purpose. The key to succeeding with this choice is planning. Don't be impulsive. For example, when Jeff Bezos quit his lucrative Wall Street job to start his new venture, he had done his research and knew exactly the risk he was taking. He has said that when Amazon was launched, he thought there was a 30% chance of success. He told his parents it was very likely they would lose all the money they were investing in his startup.

But for Bezos, there was another risk that was even greater than the financial risk he was taking. This was the risk that if he did nothing and just stayed at his secure job in finance, and years later it became clear that his idea could have succeeded, he would suffer sharp regret. He calls it his principle of regret minimization.

The future represents risk and the unknown. If you can embrace this, then your chances of working happy and having a satisfying work/life synergy increase. This brings to mind a beautiful poem by Kahlil Gibran, simply called "Fear." It's about overcoming fears, understanding our commonality, and moving forward:

Fear

It is said that before entering the sea
a river trembles with fear.

She looks back at the path she has traveled,
from the peaks of the mountains,
the long winding road crossing forests and villages.

And in front of her,
she sees an ocean so vast,
that to enter
there seems nothing more than to disappear forever.

But there is no other way.
The river cannot go back.

Nobody can go back.
To go back is impossible in existence.

The river needs to take the risk
of entering the ocean
because only then will fear disappear,
because that's where the river will know
it's not about disappearing into the ocean,
but of becoming the ocean.

IKIGAI — YOUR "LIFE-VALUE"

The idea that every person needs work and a purpose in their life has existed in many cultures.

In ancient Greece, Plato asserted that the purpose of humankind was to attain the highest form of knowledge from which all physical things sprung. With a slightly different approach, his student Aristotle proposed that the purpose of a person was to become virtuous: "Everything is done with a goal, and that goal is good."

Roman author Pliny the Elder wrote: "True glory consists in doing what deserves to be written, in writing what deserves to be read, and in so living as to make the world happier and better for our living in it."

Let's fast-forward nearly two millennia to reflect on the simple words of Robert F. Kennedy: "The purpose of life is to contribute in some way to making things better."

French culture has given us the expression "*raison d'être*," meaning "reason for being" or "reason to be." Similarly, the Japanese have a useful word for the concept of purpose: "*ikigai*," which means "life-value" in the sense of the thing that *to you* gives your life its worth.

Your *ikigai* can be found at the intersection of four personal traits:

1. What you're good at.
2. What you love.
3. What the world needs.
4. What you can be paid for.

If you think about Joe Ades, whom I profiled earlier in this chapter, his *ikigai* was deceptively simple:

1. He was good at being a salesman.
2. He loved being a salesman.
3. The world needed $5 vegetable peelers. They were genuinely useful tools.
4. His audiences were happy to buy his $5 vegetable peelers.

It may seem obvious that what you're good at should be what you love. But wait — it's really not so obvious at all. What you're *good at* is often what you've *been trained to do.* The world is full of people who have been trained in a certain skill or profession but who don't really love it and would be much happier doing something else.

Likewise, what the world needs and what you can be paid for may seem to be the same thing, but not always. For example, the world definitely needs cheap solar panels that can power an entire house and have a battery backup for nighttime and cloudy days. We're getting close to that, but we're not there yet, and you may not make much money if you try to enter that business.

Some of the current obstacles to affordable solar power for homes include the high cost of solar panels, sunlight dependency, installation challenges, space constraints, and the cost of stationary batteries for energy storage. But this is why there are often government subsidies for solar installations, so if you really love the idea of getting into the home solar industry, perhaps now is the time to do it!

Which brings us back to the question of money, which is qualification #4. If you don't care about the money or don't need the money, you can skip qualification #4. Mother Teresa forged ahead and did #1, #2, and especially #3, and didn't give much thought to the money aspect of her *ikigai*. If you want to enter the home solar panel business with the hope that someday it will be profitable without subsidies, then go for it!

Research suggests that having a strong *ikigai* will help you live longer. In 2016, Héctor Garcia co-authored *Ikigai: The Japanese Secret to a Long and Happy Life,* based in part on his work with the inhabitants of Ogimi Village on the Japanese island of Okinawa, who in the late 20th century were renowned for their longevity. His interviews with them revealed that these healthy and active seniors each had an *ikigai* they could specifically name. "When we asked what their *ikigai* was," he told *Kizuna*, "they gave us explicit answers, such as their friends, gardening, and art. Everyone knows what the source of their zest for life is and is busily engaged in it every day."[75]

The world's so-called "blue zones" are geographical areas where people live longer than the average. As identified by researchers Gianni Pes, Michel Poulain, and Dan Buettner, these five regions include Okinawa, Japan; Sardinia, Italy; Nicoya, Costa Rica; Icaria, Greece; and Loma Linda, United States. The combination of factors that make a blue zone are the ones you'd expect: a healthy diet, movement/exercise, and having friends and community. The people curate a simple life with plenty of time outdoors, enough sleep, few possessions, an active life with friends, and a light and healthy diet. To this they add a strong sense of "life value" and doing what they love, and it all adds up to a longer, happier life.

CHAPTER 10

Keep Working Happy!

LET'S IMAGINE THAT YOU'RE WORKING HAPPY and your work/life synergy is in perfect balance. You're pursuing your purpose, and you feel good about your role in the world and your contribution to it. You experience challenges in your life and work, but rather than be shaken by them, you enjoy overcoming them.

But, of course, life is nothing but change. Stress waxes and wanes. Your body ages or may suffer from disease. Tragedies loom and plans are disrupted. Even if you're pursuing the purpose for which you were made, there will be setbacks and times when you need to regroup and reaffirm your priorities and your mission.

For these times — indeed, for all times — your continued happiness and success will depend on your mental, physical, and emotional health. You're only as capable as the condition of your physical body and mind, and to perform at your very best while staying happy and avoiding getting burned out, you need to be as fit as you can be.

Here are the most important tools that you have in your kit to keep yourself working and happy.

YOUR DIET, WEIGHT, AND HEALTH

The old saying "You are what you eat" has never been truer than it is today. This is because, in the industrialized world of the 21st century, most of us have access to more food and food varieties than we can possibly consume — and we're not handling it well.

Health experts recommend that to maintain good health, women take in 2,000 calories daily and men consume 2,500 calories per day. Thanks to advanced mechanized agriculture, farmers in the United States produce food equal in value to almost 4,000 calories per day per person. This productivity is unparalleled in human history, during which regular periods of famine have been the norm.

We have a bounty of food, yet as a society, we're increasingly sedentary. We spend less time moving and more time sitting than any generation before us. We also spend more time eating. According to the United Nations (UN) Food and Agriculture Organization (FAO), in 2021, people in Europe and North America consumed an average of 3,540 calories per day. Think about it: That's nearly 50% more than we need.

The FAO indicates that African nations consume the least calories, with the number standing at 2,600, which is actually where we all should be.[76]

There are consequences to excessive eating: We're getting bigger around the waist. Health experts gauge a person's body fat by using the body mass index (BMI), which is their weight in kilograms divided by the square of height in meters. For people who aren't professional bodybuilders, a high BMI can indicate high body fat. Here's the scale:

- BMI of less than 18.5 is the underweight range.
- BMI of 18.5 to <25 is the healthy weight range.
- BMI of 25.0 to <30 is the overweight range.
- BMI of 30.0 or higher is within the obesity range.

According to the CDC, in 2017, 41.9% of the U.S. population was obese. Think about that for a moment: In 2017, nearly *half of all Americans were classified as obese*. And the rate is increasing.

Why is this a problem? Because excess fat, and obesity in particular, carries significant health risks and costs. Obesity-related conditions include heart disease, stroke, type 2 diabetes, and certain types of cancer. These "lifestyle diseases" are among the leading causes of preventable, premature death.

Research has found that among people who didn't smoke and had no apparent heart disease, those with BMIs in the healthy range of 22.5 to 24.9 were more than twice as likely to stay alive during the study period than those whose BMI was in the upper obesity range between 40 and 49.9.[77]

In 2019, the estimated annual medical cost of obesity in the United States was nearly $173 billion. Medical costs for adults with obesity were an average of $1,861 higher than medical costs for people with healthy weight.[78]

Since U.S. farmers produce so much food, you'd think that we'd be eating healthy meals. Ironically, in many areas the opposite is true. While the agricultural industry is enormous, so is the processed foods industry. Much of the food we eat is full of sugar, primarily high fructose corn syrup (HFC). While consumption has been declining — no doubt because of increasing public education and outcry — in 2019, each American consumed an average of 1.6 ounces of HFC in processed pizzas, bagels, bread, and candies daily. That does not include added sugars and other sweeteners.

As Rutgers University researchers have pointed out, a portion of the responsibility must be placed on America's food manufacturers who know how to fool health-conscious consumers. For example, one cup of Dannon Low-Fat Vanilla Yogurt contains a whopping 8.12 teaspoons of sugar, and the seemingly diet-friendly VitaminWater contains 4 teaspoons.[79]

In total, Americans consume 4.4 ounces of sugars — that's more than ¼ pound every single day.

The twin challenges of being overweight and eating too much sugar affect your ability to work happy. The sequence of cause and effect is simple: The more sugar you eat, the more depressed you may become, and in an attempt to "lift your spirits," you may consume even more sugar, making your depression worse and your weight soar in a vicious cycle.

One scientific study found "overwhelming evidence" indicating that "sucrose consumption results in pathophysiological consequences such as morphological neuronal changes, altered emotional processing, and modified behavior."[80] A 2022 study found that among obese adults, a high intake of total sugar was associated with "increased odds of clinically relevant depressive symptoms."[81]

To keep working happy, one of the first things you can do is eliminate as much sugar as you can from your diet, eat healthy foods, and keep your weight within the normal range. The same applies for all the other contaminants we put into our bodies: alcohol, tobacco, and recreational drugs. Limit your alcohol consumption, quit smoking, and be very careful with drugs like marijuana, which is now legal in many states. Don't use *any* of these substances at work, only at home, if you must. You'll think more clearly, be less stressed at work, and live a longer, more productive life.

Let's talk about *dieting,* as in following a specified program to reduce calorie intake in order to lose weight. In America, our pursuit of weight loss has led to the creation of a vast diet-foods industry that is today valued at $200 billion, and as the rate of adult obesity climbs, the diet foods industry is expected to continue to grow to nearly $300 billion by 2027. It's a multifaceted market with five segments:

1. **Better-for-you (BFY).** This is the biggest segment and includes supermarket foods that are marketed as "healthier choices." These foods may be described as being low in salt and sugar, high in fiber, and/or with added vitamins. They're not specifically low-calorie diet foods.

2. **Meal replacement.** This "healthy" alternative to meals contains all the required nutrients and is low in calories and high in protein. The powder segment of meal replacement consists of powders added to milk or water to make a "meal" or shake and rules the meal replacement market. The market size was $11.9 billion in 2021 and is projected to reach $15.5 billion by 2026.

3. **Weight-loss supplement.** This market consists of pills, capsules, powders, drinks, and energy bars that contain vitamins, minerals, herbs, and other ingredients purported to promote weight loss. These supplements claim to boost metabolism and thermogenesis while decreasing macronutrient absorption, hunger, body fat, and weight.

4. **Green tea.** Increasingly popular among millennials as a healthy, organic, and plant-based beverage, green tea is now consumed all over the world. Green tea claims a long list of health advantages, including weight loss, detoxification, and more.

To this category, you might add substances that purport to boost metabolism, such as cayenne pepper (not to be added to your green tea but used as a separate item). The active ingredient in cayenne pepper is capsaicin, which is also found in other types of peppers. Research suggests that capsaicin is a thermogenic chemical that may help speed up metabolism and decrease appetite. Other substances that have the same effect include caffeine, L-carnitine, chromium picolinate, and conjugated linoleic acid (CLA).

5. **Low-calorie sweeteners.** These are sugar substitutes that have low-calorie levels and do not raise blood glucose levels. They're aimed at consumers, particularly those at risk for diabetes, looking to reduce their sugar consumption. Some common types of these sweeteners are aspartame, acesulfame-K, saccharin, sucralose, neotame, and advantame.

6. **Weight-loss drugs.** These include a compound called semaglutide, which is sold under the brand names Ozempic, Wegovy, and Rybelsus. Developed by Novo Nordisk in 2012, it's an antidiabetic medication used for the treatment of type 2 diabetes as well as an anti-obesity medication for long-term weight management. It works as an appetite suppressant and helps control blood sugar levels by prompting the body to release insulin.

This growing market joins companies like Weight Watchers, Nutri-System, Noom, and Jenny Craig that provide a complete diet plan, often with prepared meals sent to your door. Memberships in weight loss programs are dominated by women; an estimated 90% of Weight Watchers members are women.

If all else fails, you can always undergo a type of bariatric surgery, which includes gastric bypass, sleeve gastrectomy, gastric band, and duodenal switch. Targeted mainly at patients who are obese, the number of surgeries performed has increased by 10% in the last decade alone. In various ways, this surgery reduces the size of the stomach and for obese patients has been an effective weight loss technique.

As you can see, we Americans spend billions of dollars to consume more food and then spend billions more to try to lose the weight we gain by eating so much.

If the idea is to help you lose weight so that you don't need to pay to diet anymore, why is the American diet industry so successful and profitable?

Because their products don't work — and yet we keep buying them.

According to *Scientific American*, research suggests that roughly 80% of people who lose weight will not maintain that degree of weight loss for 12 months; dieters regain, on average, more than half of what they lose within two years.[82]

The more diet attempts you make, the more likely you are to gain weight in the future. As *Psychology Today* pointed out, most diets are rigid and unsustainable. On average, weight loss attempts last just four weeks for women and six weeks for men before they give up and go back to their regular eating habits.

To get you to eat less, diets usually demonize a particular food group, such as carbohydrates or fats. Foods with "too many carbs," "too much fat," or "too many calories" are seen as "bad." You count the calories you consume, which piles on a big load of guilt if you slip up.[83]

The number of types of diets is overwhelming. The Paleo dieters say we should eat like our caveman ancestors did, when the average life expectancy was about 30 years. The Atkins Diet allows protein and fat, but few carbohydrates. The South Beach diet went a step further and advocated high protein, low fat, and low carbs. Vegan diets eliminate animal protein. The Zone diet specifies a diet strictly composed of 30% lean protein, 30% healthy fat, and 40% high-fiber carbs. And on they go....

Astounding, isn't it? While these diets may have a theoretical basis for efficacy, in the real world they often fall short because, for various reasons, the people who might benefit from them cannot stick with them.

In contrast to all the costly pills, plans, and procedures, here's a weight-control secret that's both free and highly effective:

It's easier to eat *nothing* for a short period of time every day than to consume low-calorie meals and snacks to "curb your hunger" or get you "over the hump." This is because low-calorie meals leave you feeling unsatisfied and quickly feeling hungry again. If you surrender and have a snack in the afternoon, it will stimulate your appetite and make you want to eat more. The constant feeling of hunger is exhausting and quickly wears you down.

The best way to maintain a healthy weight is to eat the way the human body has been designed to consume food for thousands of years: *intermittent fasting*. To be clear, we're *not* talking about unhealthy self-starvation, such as anorexia, which is a serious eating disorder. We're talking about mindful eating and ensuring the stomach is empty for several hours per day, which is the way the digestive system is designed to operate at its highest efficiency.

Just eat healthy foods: whole-grain carbs, protein, and fat. Minimize processed food products. Enjoy your meal. Then eat *nothing* until your next meal. No snacks, no Starbucks, no candy bars. Just water or plain tea. And one more thing: Eat nothing for a 12-hour period every day. That should be easy because it's roughly the overnight period from dinner (7 p.m.) to breakfast (7 a.m.). Eat three normal meals within 12 hours and abstain from eating for the next 12 hours. Of course, if you prefer, you can fast for any length of time, with 24 hours generally being the longest safe period.

Do you want to know something interesting? As recently as 1960, the American population weighed much less. The average adult woman weighed 140 pounds in 1960, and by 2010, her weight had increased to 166.2 pounds. The average man weighed 166.3 pounds in 1960 and is now up to 195.5 pounds. That's an average increase of over four pounds per decade![84]

This is because we eat too much and move too little. It's just that simple.

By the way, beware of food additives that may be harmful to your health. The European Union prohibits or restricts many food additives that have been linked to cancer, while in the United States, they are still allowed in bread, cookies, soft drinks, and other processed foods. Many European countries limit the cultivation and import of genetically modified foods and ban the use of several drugs that are permitted for use in farm animals in the United States. These substances include potassium bromate and azodicarbonamide (ADA),

BHA and BHT, brominated vegetable oil (BVO), red food dye No. 40 and yellow food dyes No. 5 and No. 6, and many veterinary drugs.[85]

Try mindful eating. Eat slowly, chew thoroughly, remove distractions, and stop eating when you're full. Eat only when you're hungry and avoid "recreational eating" and eating to soothe an emotional issue. It's a more holistic approach to what you put into your body and much easier than fad diets. You'll gradually lose weight, you won't feel deprived, and you'll be better prepared to work happy.

MEDITATION

One of the most time-honored and successful methods of de-stressing at work, at home, or just about anywhere is meditation.

Meditation is simply any practice in which an individual focuses the mind on a particular object, thought, or activity to achieve a mentally clear and emotionally calm and stable state that is free of judgment, anxiety, or action. The practice of meditation has been studied and recorded for thousands of years and is deeply woven into many religions and cultures, including Buddhism, Hinduism, Taoism, Jainism, Judaism, Islam, and Christianity. In America, the modern interest in meditation began in the 1960s with two global events.

The first was the rise of communism, which drove many Asian spiritual teachers to seek refuge in the West. Notably, in March 1959, the Dalai Lama was forced to leave Tibet to begin a permanent exile in India, thereby thrusting him into the spotlight as he campaigned for Tibetan freedom at the United Nations. Had he not been persecuted, he may never have come to such prominence in the West.

The other event was the Baby Boomer wave of young people in Europe and America. In the mid- and late-1960s, the U.S. government was waging war in Vietnam that was deeply unpopular among this enormous generation of draft-age students. They started looking for alternative sources of spiritual guidance just at the time when Eastern teachers were gaining prominence.

A watershed moment came in February 1968, when the Beatles traveled to Rishikesh in northern India to participate in a training course in Transcendental Meditation at the ashram of Maharishi

Mahesh Yogi. The visit received widespread media attention, helped change Western attitudes about Indian spirituality, and validated the study of Transcendental Meditation.

The useful thing about meditation is that while you can subscribe to any one of many traditions and practices, you can do it however you like. You can make it a lifelong study or just dabble at your own speed. While adherents to the various methods may dispute whether a particular practice is legitimate, at the end of the day, the choice is yours.

The only real requirement is that you be in an environment in which you may meditate undisturbed by other people and their activities. Most people think of meditating at home, in the morning or evening, but if you have a quiet place at work, you can do it there. I know a man who used to work in a factory. Every few hours, there was a mandatory break, and the line would pause. All the workers would hurry outside for their break, leaving the factory floor virtually deserted. He'd sit on a pile of boxes and meditate for 10 minutes. He was roused from his meditative state by the ringing of the bell. Those few minutes helped him to clear his mind and prepare for the next sprint.

Places you can meditate include:

- **A special meditation room in your home or at work.** Big companies such as Salesforce, Nike, Pearson, Google, Yahoo, and HBO have designated official meditation spaces in their corporate offices. Steve Jobs was a strong advocate of meditation, and at Apple, he introduced 30-minute daily meditation breaks and had meditation rooms built throughout their offices worldwide.[86]
- **On the banks of a pond, lake, or river, or by a fountain.** The gentle sound of running or lapping water facilitates meditation. It calms the mind and helps it to remain in the present moment. It also suggests the impermanence of thought and that troublesome things will come and go.
- **Parks and gardens.** Especially if you live in a city, finding a green spot with trees overhead and grass underfoot can provide a welcome change of atmosphere. Fresh air and a new aware-

ness of the interconnectedness and harmony with other living beings make it easy to slip into a meditative state. Grounding and coming into physical contact with the earth offers significant benefits for both mental and physical health.

- **Rooftop or balcony.** Even in a busy building, it may be possible to find some tranquility by stepping out onto a balcony or going up to the roof. In 1964, a hit song called "Up on the Roof" by The Drifters captured this feeling wonderfully; it extolled the pleasures of getting "above it all" even in the busy city:

  "When this old world starts getting me down
  And people are just too much for me to face
  I climb way up to the top of the stairs
  And all my cares just drift right into space
  On the roof, it's peaceful as can be
  And there the world below can't bother me..."[87]

- **Sacred spaces.** Whether or not you're religious, the quiet solitude offered by churches, temples, and mosques encourages introspection and communion. Look for a sacred place — even one in nature — with an atmosphere of serenity that's a good fit for your meditation practice.

No matter how or where you do it, or even what you call it, taking a few minutes to calm your mind and let go of burdensome thoughts can help keep you working happy.

EXERCISE

Just as our diets have become challenging in our new world of processed foods and 24-hour calorie delivery, so has our physical fitness. Americans spend more time sitting in one place than ever before in human history. We sit in our cars. We sit at our desks. We sit on our sofas and watch other people play sports on TV. We sit and eat.

The U.S. Department of Health and Human Services recommends healthy adults spend at least 150 minutes per week — about 20 minutes a day — doing moderate-intensity aerobic exercise, and at least two days per week doing muscle-strengthening activities.[88]

According to the CDC, more than 60% of American adults do not engage in the recommended amount of activity; approximately 25% of adults are not active at all. As we know from the previous section on weight and diet, we're increasingly heavy. The heavier we get and closer to obesity, the less likely we are to want to exercise, thus compounding our problem.

A 2021 survey of American adults found that a plurality (39.4%) reported *never* working out or exercising vigorously in a given week. Despite the ongoing awareness of the state of our health, and despite physical exercise being one of the best predictors of health and longevity, many of us are foregoing physical activity in our day-to-day lives.[89]

As the CDC advises, the health benefits of physical fitness are many and include:

- **Brain health.** The benefits of physical activity on brain health include improved thinking and cognition and reduced short-term feelings of anxiety. It can help keep thinking, learning, and judgment skills sharp as we age, reduce our risk of depression and anxiety, and help us sleep better.
- **Body health.** Getting at least 150 minutes a week of moderate physical activity can put us at a lower risk for heart disease and stroke, two leading causes of death in the United States. It can also lower blood pressure and improve cholesterol levels.
- **Reduction in type 2 diabetes and metabolic syndrome.** Regular physical activity can reduce the risk of developing type 2 diabetes as well as metabolic syndrome, which is a combination of high blood pressure, too much fat around the waist, low high-density lipoproteins (HDL) "good" cholesterol, high triglycerides, or high blood sugar.
- **Reduction in cancer development.** Physical activity lowers the risk of developing several common cancers.
- **Stronger bones and muscles.** Weight training can help maintain or increase muscle mass and strength. Older adults in particular can experience reduced muscle mass and muscle strength and should exercise regularly to maintain strong bones as well as mobility and balance.

- **Longer life.** Something as simple as walking for 15 minutes every day or just walking more frequently throughout the day can add years to your life. As *The Lancet*, a prominent medical journal, reported, taking more steps per day has been associated with a progressively lower risk of all-cause mortality. Counting the number of steps per day is a simple and easily interpreted metric that can enhance doctor–patient and public health communication for monitoring and promoting a person's physical activity.[90]

LIFELONG LEARNING

Back in the 1960s and 1970s, many people had the idea that you went to school only when you were young. At a certain point, you'd reach your educational objective — bachelor's degree, master's degree, or even doctorate — and then you'd stop going to school and enter the workforce. If you were a woman, you typically got married and had a family. A man might go back to earn a professional degree, such as an MBA, but the idea that adults would attend college in any great numbers was unimaginable. College was for kids, and while you would certainly want to keep up with current events, as an adult your job was to work until you retired. If you stayed at one company for your entire career, there was no particular reason to go back to school because you could learn on the job.

But times have changed. Companies became less loyal, more people kept working later in life, the pace of innovation and disruption accelerated, and more women embarked on professional careers. These changes did two things to workers: They intensified the chances of getting burned out on the job and, for many workers, they made it more urgent to access new educational opportunities. A new certification or degree, or even coursework, became an asset on a resume and simplified job changes or career advancement.

The Great Recession of 2008 promoted the growth of adult education, as people realized additional education could improve their chances of landing employment. In 1970, the number of adults aged 20 or older going back to school was about 5.7 million. By 2024, it's expected to reach 18.5 million — over three times the number.[91]

The old stereotype of the fresh-faced college kid or co-ed (as female students were unflatteringly called) is giving way to a new reality: According to the Lumina Foundation, 38% of undergraduate students are older than 25, 58% are working while enrolled in college, and 26% are raising children. To provide a better life for themselves and their family, the typical student today must balance life, school, and work.[92]

Online learning has made going back to school even easier. Business management firm McKinsey and Company reported that in the decade from 2011 to 2021, the number of students reached by massive open online courses (MOOCs) increased from 300,000 to 220 million. These are online courses aimed at unlimited participation and open access via the internet.

During the seven years between 2012 and 2019, the number of hybrid and distance-only students at traditional universities increased by 36%, and in 2020, spurred by the COVID pandemic, growth rapidly accelerated that by an additional 92%.[93]

New course offerings are blurring the lines between degree and non-degree learning, creating a new category of educational consumers. Ordinary people are developing a keen interest in courses in high-demand areas such as data analytics and user experience design and have caused significant gains in enrollment. These programs give prospective learners cost-effective, easy-to-access options outside a degree program. Meanwhile, traditional digital education providers that are primarily degree-focused are now including such offerings to compete and grow in the online education space.

You can go back to school at any age.

Nola Ochs, who died in 2016 at the age of 105, was a woman from Jetmore, Kansas. In 2007, at age 95, she graduated from Fort Hays State University with a bachelor of general studies degree. She was certified by Guinness World Records as the oldest person in the world to become a college graduate. To make it even better, she graduated alongside her 21-year-old granddaughter, Alexandra Ochs.

In 2016, however, her record was surpassed by Shigemi Hirata, who received a bachelor of arts degree from the Kyoto University of Art and Design in Kyoto, Japan, on March 19, 2016. Born in 1919, he was age 96 years and 200 days old when he received his diploma after 11 years of study.[94]

In-person or online continuing education classes allow workers to slow down and gain the insights needed to be more productive in their work. The more education and experience they gain, the less likely they'll experience burnout. Learning to become better at whatever you do is an ongoing process.

Physicians, pharmacists, and real estate agents are required to continue their education. Mandatory continuing education (MCE) is often specified by the regulatory standards of the U.S. Department of Labor's Occupational Safety and Health Administration (OSHA), the U.S. Environmental Protection Agency (EPA), and the U.S. Department of Transportation (DOT). MCE comprises the ongoing professional development courses taken within one's professional field to demonstrate current competence and maintain certification or licensure.

Physicians are required to take continuing medical education courses (CMEs); nurses and other allied health professionals are usually required to acquire a certain number of continuing education units (CEUs); certified safety professionals need CEUs; certified industrial hygienists (CIHs) accumulate certification maintenance points (CMs); the list goes on.

It's crucial that through continuing education, we all continue to learn how to best serve our profession, our customers, and ourselves while staying current with the most up-to-date knowledge.

VOLUNTEER IN SERVICE TO OTHERS

At first, volunteering may seem to be a contradiction in the sense that if you're feeling burned out at work, why would you want to do more work somewhere else for free? Because being burned out at work can mean many things. It may mean that you're just tired of doing the same thing day after day, but for some reason, you don't want to give up your job. The job may provide you with security, it may pay well, or it may be basically what you want to do with your life, but you need more stimulation and challenge.

And it also depends on what you mean by "work." Look at it

this way: There are a total of 168 hours in a week. Let's say you work at your regular job 40 hours a week. That's eight hours a day, five days a week.

That leaves 128 hours in your week. If you sleep eight hours a night, that's 56 hours per week, leaving 72 hours. Give yourself four hours a day for commuting, eating, and self-care, which leaves 44 hours a week for everything else.

You have 44 hours a week to do something. Anything!

You could work a second job, either full-time or part-time. According to the Bureau of Labor Statistics, more than 400,000 Americans work two full-time jobs. Many more people work a full-time job plus a part-time job. As of September 2022, 4.9% of all the more than 164 million U.S. workers, or over 7.7 million people, held two or more job positions.[95] If this is what you need to do, you may be excused from also doing volunteer work.

You could sit and watch TV. Statistics show the average American watches about 18 hours of TV per week.

You could read. The average is about two hours per week.

You could pursue a hobby like golf, or gardening, or arts and crafts.

You could meditate or just stare off into space.

No matter what it is, during those 44 hours that you're not working your primary job, you're going to be doing *something*. Why not allocate some of the 44 hours to something that you enjoy, that enriches you, and helps other people? If you like doing it, then it won't seem like "work." It will be a pleasant and productive activity.

For Americans who like to volunteer, the government-sponsored AmeriCorps divides volunteering into two categories: formal and informal. Formal volunteering is provided through established charitable and nonprofit organizations, while informal volunteering means assisting others outside of an organizational context.

AmeriCorps reported that between September 2020 and 2021, an estimated 23.2% of Americans, or more than 60.7 million people, volunteered with recognized organizations. They contributed an estimated 4.1 billion hours of their time with an economic value of $122.9 billion. Meanwhile, during the same period, nearly 51%

of Americans, or 124.7 million people, informally helped their neighbors.[96]

Volunteerism has long been woven into the fabric of American life. As a frontier nation in the 18th and 19th centuries, while "every man for himself" may have been a romantic notion, in reality, people came together to solve problems and help each other. This commitment to volunteerism has been a hallmark of American civic life ever since Benjamin Franklin formed the first volunteer fire department in 1736, and in fact, today, around 70% of American firefighters are volunteers. Many American militias during the Revolutionary War were comprised of volunteers, while non-combatant civilian volunteers contributed money and services to the effort.

Writing about his travels through the United States in the 1830s, the French political scientist Alexis de Tocqueville frequently noted Americans' willingness to form voluntary civil associations and was impressed by the newly independent Americans' desire to come together with their friends and neighbors to accomplish community and personal goals. In his classic *Democracy in America,* he wrote:

"In the United States, as soon as several inhabitants have taken an opinion or an idea they wish to promote in society, they seek each other out and unite together once they have made contact. From that moment, they are no longer isolated but have become a power seen from afar whose activities serve as an example and whose words are heeded."[97]

This may surprise you, but while we may assume that people who do not work or who are retired have the most time to volunteer, in 2015, the Bureau of Labor Statistics found that employed people ages 35 to 44 were most likely to volunteer. Of those who volunteered, 33% helped a religious organization, while 25% chose educational or youth service organizations.

And by the way, the median number of volunteer hours is 52 per year. That happens to be exactly one hour per week.[98]

Volunteering in service to others, whether in a formal job-like setting or informally, can be spiritually and emotionally uplifting. Instead of spending your free time in activities that benefit no one —

including yourself — you're helping to make someone else's life better. As an added bonus, when you volunteer at a place that is neither your home nor your workplace, you will refresh your mind and heart and make it easier to take another five-day, nine-to-five plunge into your regular job.

Thank You!

Thank you for reading this book.

I hope it has provided you with fresh insights into the growing problem of job and career burnout, which can affect anyone's life, including yours. To be armed with knowledge about the problem is to be halfway to winning the battle, and ultimately, to succeed requires practical and actionable ideas, which this book has endeavored to deliver. If you're feeling burned out with your job, take it step by step:

1. Think about exactly what's causing your burnout. It could be multiple factors. Be honest and avoid preconceptions. If necessary, make a list.

2. Figure out what you can do to turn burnout into joy. You can change your environment or change yourself. Those are your two choices. You may need to do both.

3. Take action! Make the changes you've envisioned. Be fearless. Embrace the future. Think about how you can help other people to lead better lives. Try not to worry about the money; you may be surprised to know how quickly money flows toward those who believe in themselves and are engaged in helping a neighbor.

I'd love to hear from you!

LinkedIn: https://www.linkedin.com/in/roger-kapoor/
Facebook: https://www.facebook.com/Rogerkapoormd/
X: @rogerkapoormd
Instagram: rogerkapoormd

References

1. Kane CK. Recent Changes in Physician Practice Arrangements: Private Practice Dropped to Less Than 50 Percent of Physicians in 2020. *Policy Research Perspectives*. AMA. 2021. https://www.ama-assn.org/system/files/2021-05/2020-prp-physician-practice-arrangements.pdf

2. O'Kane C. Nurse Who Raised Concern About Lack of PPE Died From Coronavirus — Just Days Before Her Planned Retirement. CBS News. April 27, 2020. https://www.cbsnews.com/news/nurse-died-coronavirus-kansas-city-missouri-celia-yap-banago-ppe-protest/

3. Silver-Greenberg J, Drucker J, Enrich D. Hospitals Got Bailouts and Furloughed Thousands While Paying CEOs Millions. *The New York Times*. June 8, 2020. https://www.nytimes.com/2020/06/08/business/hospitals-bailouts-ceo-pay.html

4. Chapman B. Hospital Cleaners for Private Healthcare Giant "Forced to Work without PPE or Proper Training." *The Independent*. February 15, 2020. https://www.independent.co.uk/news/business/hospital-cleaners-covid-ppe-safety-b2014576.html

5. Morgenson G, Schecter A, McFadden C. Roaches in the Operating Room: Doctors at HCA Hospital in Florida Say Patient Care Has Suffered From Cost Cutting. NBC News. February 15, 2023. https://www.nbcnews.com/health/health-care/roaches-operating-room-hca-hospital-florida-rcna69563

6. ShiftNursing. How Burnout Impacts Nursing: Before, During, and After COVID-19. Shift. April 25, 2020. https://www.shiftnursing.com/articles/nurse-burnout/

7. American Nurses Foundation. American Nurses Foundation Releases Comprehensive Survey About Nurses. Press Release. American Nurses Foundation. March 10, 2021. https://www.nursingworld.org/news/news-releases/2021/american-nurses-foundation-releases-comprehensive-survey-about-nurses/

8. Draze L. COVID-19 and PTSD in Frontline Nurses. American Nurse. October 4, 2022. ANA. https://www.myamericannurse.com/covid-19-and-ptsd-in-frontline-nurses/

9. Staff. World's Oldest Practicing Doctor Offers Advice on Staying Mentally Sharp. Psychiatrist.com. May 16, 2023. https://www.psychiatrist.com/news/worlds-oldest-practicing-doctor-offers-advice-on-staying-mentally-sharp/#:~:text=Howard%20Tucker%2C%20MD%2C%20a%20neurologist,help%20hold%20off%20cognitive%20decline.

10. NurseHack4Health. NurseHack4Health Pitch-A-Thon. https://www.youtube.com/watch?v=tl36j3_kzlo&list=PLZhOr4T9V2JP3uqJNZDK-_HJqp0NLfh6P

11. Arnold C. Former Wells Fargo Employees Describe Toxic Sales Culture, Even at HQ. NPR. October 4, 2016. https://www.npr.org/2016/10/04/496508361/former-wells-fargo-employees-describe-toxic-sales-culture-even-at-hq

12. Kalpan A, Nguyen V, Godie M. Overworked, Understaffed: Pharmacists Say Industry in Crisis Puts Patient Safety at Risk. NBC News. March 16, 2021. https://www.nbcnews.com/health/health-care/overworked-understaffed-pharmacists-say-industry-crisis-puts-patient-safety-risk-n1261151

13. Abbruzzese J, Holmes A, Martinez D, Ingram D. Google Walkout: Employees Stage Protest Over Handling of Sexual Harassment by Executives. NBC News. November 1, 2018. https://www.nbcnews.com/tech/tech-news/google-employees-begin-walkout-over-handling-sexual-misconduct-executives-n929696

14. Huddleston T. Founder of 1-800-GOT-JUNK? Dropped out of College to Haul Junk – Now, He's Eyeing a Billion-Dollar Business. CNBC. August 1, 2020. https://www.cnbc.com/2020/08/01/how-the-1-800-got-junk-founder-became-a-multimillionaire.html#:~:text=billion%2Ddollar%20business-,Founder%20of%201%2D800%2DGOT%2DJUNK%3F,eyeing%20a%20billion%2Ddollar%20business&text=Tom%20Huddleston%20Jr.&text=Inspiration%20can%20strike%20at%20any%20moment.

15. The Bench Team. How Brian Scudamore Fired Everyone and Saved 1-800-Got-Junk? Bench.co. November 14, 2018. https://bench.co/blog/small-business-stories/brian-scudamore/

16. Glassdoor. 1-800-GOT-JUNK? Overview. Glassdoor.com. https://www.glassdoor.com/Overview/Working-at-1-800-GOT-JUNK-EI_IE22742.11,25.htm

17. Gates B. What I Learned from Warren Buffett. *Harvard Business Review*. January-February 1996. https://hbr.org/1996/01/what-i-learned-from-warren-buffett

18. Elkins K. Warren Buffett Spends 8 Hours a Week Playing the "Only Game" at Which He May Be Better Than Bill Gates. CNBC. February 25, 2019. https://www.cnbc.com/2019/02/25/warren-buffett-plays-bridge-8-hours-a-week-and-can-beat-bill-gates.html#:~:text=Buffett%2C%20who%20is%2C%20at%2088,hand%2C%E2%80%9D%20he%20told%20Heath.

19. Coffee K. With Musicians — and Even Warren Buffett — The Ukelele Is Making It Big. *Omaha World-Herald*. October 16, 2019. https://omaha.com/lifestyles/with-musicians-and-even-warren-buffett-the-ukulele-is-making/article_9616a5a4-7ac8-5b04-9150-808022f92df9.html?mode=jqm

20. GuruFocus. Warren Buffett: Take a Job That You Love. Nasdaq. April 22, 2016. https://www.nasdaq.com/articles/warren-buffett-take-job-you-love-2016-04-22

21. Holt-Lunstad J, Smith TB, Layton JB. Social Relationships and Mortality Risk: A Meta-analytic Review. *PLoS Med*. 2010;7(7): e1000316. https://doi.org/10.1371/journal.pmed.1000316

22. American Sleep Apnea Association. The State of Sleep Health in America 2023. Sleephealth.org. https://www.sleephealth.org/sleep-health/the-state-of-sleephealth-in-america/#:~:text=In%20America%2C%2070%25%20of%20adults,report%20insufficient%20sleep%20every%20

night.&text=It%20is%20estimated%20that%20sleep,all%20ages%20 and%20socioeconomic%20classes.

23. Colton HR and Altevogt MB, eds. Sleep Disorders and Sleep Deprivation: An Unmet Public Health Problem. Board on Health Sciences Policy. Washington, DC: National Academies Press, 2006.

24. Branson R. Delegating vs D-I-Y. *The Star*. November 30, 2015. https://www. thestar.com.my/metro/smebiz/columns/2015/11/30/delegating-vs-diy/

25. Blum LD. Physicians' Goodness and Guilt — Emotional Challenges of Practicing Medicine. *JAMA Intern Med*. 2019:179(5):607–608. https:// jamanetwork.com/journals/jamainternalmedicine/article-abstract/2729746

26. Kalmoe MC, Chapman MB, Gold JA, Giedinghagen AM. Physician Suicide: A Call to Action. *MoMed*. 2019;116(3):211–216. https://www.ncbi.nlm.nih. gov/pmc/articles/PMC6690303/

27. Quittner J. 1999 Person of the Year. Jeff Bezos Biography. *TIME*. https:// web.archive.org/web/20000408032804/http://www.time.com/time/poy/ bezos5.html

28. Locke T. This Employee's Suggestion to Jeff Bezos Doubled Amazon's Productivity in Its First Month. CNBC. January 7, 2020. https://www.cnbc. com/2020/01/07/this-doubled-jeff-bezos-productivity-in-the-first-month-of- amazon.html

29. Kish M. *Nike Court Records Detail Sexual Harrassment, Toxic Workplace Claims. Business Insider. December 2022.* https://www.businessinsider.com/ nike-court-records-detail-sexual-harassment-toxic-workplace-claims-2022-12

30. Rousmaniere D. What Everyone Should Know About Managing Up. *Harvard Business Review*. January 23, 2015. https://hbr.org/2015/01/ what-everyone-should-know-about-managing-up

31. Culture Amp. Guide to Managing Up: What It Means and Why It's Important. CultureAmp.com. July 26, 2023. https://www.cultureamp.com/ blog/managing-up-importance

32. Bratskeir K. How to Find Work-Life Balance in a High- Pressure Job. WeWork. September 5, 2019. https://www. wework.com/ideas/professional-development/creativity-culture/ how-to-find-work-life-balance-in-a-high-pressure-job

33. NASA. She Was a Computer When Computers Wore Skirts. NASA News. August 26, 2008. https://www.nasa.gov/centers/langley/news/researchernews/ rn_kjohnson.html

34. Hartmans A. Tim Cook's Rise to the Head of Apple. Business Insider. January 13, 2024.

35. Robert Half. Nearly One-Quarter of Workers Have Left a Job Due to a Bad Commute, According to Robert Half Survey. Press Release. Robert Half. September 24, 2018. https://press.roberthalf.com/2018-09-24-Nearly -One-Quarter-Of-Workers-Have-Left-A-Job-Due-To-A-Bad-Commute- According-To-Robert-Half-Survey

36. U.S. Census Bureau. Average Travel Time To Work. U.S. Census Bureau.

2022. https://www.census.gov/search-results.html?q=commute&p age=1&stateGeo=none&searchtype=web&cs sp=SERP

37. Stillman J. Your Terrible Commute Is Making You Dumber, New Study Finds. Inc.com. August 1, 2017. https://www.inc.com/jessica-stillman/your-terrible-commute-is-making-you-dumber-new-stu.html

38. Christian TJ. Opportunity Costs Surrounding Exercise and Dietary Behaviors: Quantifying Trade-offs Between Commuting Time and Health-Related Activities. SSRN. October 21, 2009. https://ssrn.com/ abstract=1490117.

39. Reed B. Four-Day Working Week Would Slash UK Carbon Footprint, Report Says. *The Guardian*. May 27, 2021. https://www.theguardian. com/environment/2021/may/27/four-day-working-week-would-slash-uk -carbon-footprint-report

40. Gallup. State of the American Workplace. Gallup. 2017. https://www. gallup.com/workplace/238085/state-american-workplace-report-2017. aspx?thank-you-report-form=1

41. Sinha R. How to Deal with a Jealous Manager. *Harvard Business Review*. December 18, 2020. https://hbr.org/2020/12/ how-to-deal-with-a-jealous-manager

42. Gallup. State of the American Workplace. Gallup. 2017. https://www. gallup.com/workplace/238085/state-american-workplace-report-2017. aspx?thank-you-report-form=1

43. Glassdoor. Job Expectations Graph. Glassdoor.com. August 2, 2018. https:// www.glassdoor.com/employers/app/uploads/sites/2/2018/08/GD-Survey-Job-Expectations.png

44. Glassdoor. Top Companies for Work/Life Balance. Glassdoor.com. https:// www.glassdoor.com/Explore/top-companies-work-life-balance_IF.14,31_ IFID104.htm

45. McGrew S. Beloved Grocery in Southeast Wisconsin Retires After 50 Years. TMJ4 News. December 30, 2022. https://www.tmj4.com/news/local-news/ beloved-grocer-in-southeast-wisconsin-retires-after-50-years

46. Montag A. Jay Leno Learned This Life Lesson from a Pair of Myster Underwear He Found Working at McDonald's. CNBC. May 7, 2018. https:// www.cnbc.com/2018/05/07/what-working-at-mcdonalds-taught-jay-leno-about-success.html

47. Goh ZK. Vera Want Talks About Her Olympics Ambitions. International Olympic Committee News. November 3, 2020. https://olympics.com/en/ news/vera-wang-talks-about-her-olympics-ambitions

48. Fashion Elite. Vera Wang. FashionElite.com. https://fashionelite.com/profile/ vera-wang/

49. Beard A. Life's Work: An Interview with Vera Wang. *Harvard Business Review*. July-August 2019.. https://hbr.org/2019/07/lifes-work-an-interview -with-vera-wang

50. Erenhouse R. Today's Migrant. Western Union. May 2022. https://corporate. westernunion-microsites.com/wp-content/uploads/2022/05/Todays-Migrant-All-Countries-1.pdf

51. Lee LO, James P, Zevon ES, Kubzansky LD. Optimism Is Associated with Exceptional Longevity in 2 Epidemiologic Cohorts of Men and Women. *Proceedings of the National Academy of Sciences.* August 26, 2019. https:// www.pnas.org/doi/full/10.1073/pnas.1900712116

52. Chopik WJ, Oh J, Kim ES, Schwaba T, Kramer MD, et al. Changes in Optimism and Pessimism in Response to Life Events: Evidence From Three Large Panel Studies. J Research in Personality. October 2020;88: 103985. https://doi.org/10.1016/j.jrp.2020.103985.

53. DiSC. What Is DiSC? discprofile.com https://www.discprofile.com/ what-is-disc

54. The Franklin Institute. Edison's Lightbulb. https://www.fi.edu/history -resources/edisons-lightbulb

55. Leone D. Did You Know the Pre-Flight Checklist Was First Introduced by Boeing Following the 1935 Crash of the Prototype B-17? The Aviation Geek Club. July 24, 2022. https://theaviationgeekclub.com/did-you-know-the-pre-flight-checklist-was-first-introduced-by-boeing-following-the-1935-crash-of-the-prototype-b-17-then-known-as-the-model-299/

56. Screen Education. Screen Education's "Digital Distraction & Workplace Safety" Survey Finds US Employees Distracted 2.5 Hours Each Workday By Digital Content Unrelated to Their Jobs. News Release. Screen Education. August 31, 2020. t https://www.prnewswire.com/news-releases/ screen-educations-smartphone-distraction--workplace-safety-survey-finds-us-employees-distracted-2-5-hours-each-workday-by-digital-content-unrelat-ed-to-their-jobs-301120969.html

57. Care New England. 8 Ways Your Phone Can Affect Your Mental Health. Blog. Butler Hospital. January 14, 2022. https://www.butler.org/blog/ phone-affecting-your-mental-health

58. Masih N. Tired of After-Work Emails and Calls? In These Countries They're Outlawed. *The Washington Post.* February 1, 2023. https://www. washingtonpost.com/business/2023/02/01/right-to-disconnect-laws/

59. Deloitte. 2023 Travel Industry Outlook. Deloitte. 2023. https://www2. deloitte.com/us/en/pages/consumer-business/articles/travel-hospitality-industry-outlook.html

60. Liu G. "Workcations" Aren't an Escape. They're Practice. *The Atlantic.* April 21, 2022. The Atlantic. https://www.theatlantic.com/culture/archive/2022/04/ covid-workcation-remote-work-life-balance/629605/

61. Sonnentag S. 2012 Psychological Detachment From Work During Leisure Time: The Benefits of Mentally Disengaging From Work. *Current Directions in Psychological Science.* 2012:21(2):114–118. https://doi. org/10.1177/0963721411434979

62. Center for Economic and Policy Research. U.S. Only Advanced Economy

That Does Not Guarantee Paid Vacation or Holidays. News Release. Center for Economic and Policy Research. https://cepr.net/documents/publications/nvn-summary.pdf

63. EZcater. The Lunch Report. EZcater. https://1703639.fs1. hubspotusercontent-na1.net/hubfs/1703639/TheLunchReport_Food ImprovesProductivity_July_2022.pdf

64. Ivie D. SNL's Brutally Honest Tour Guide Wants to Temper Vacation Expectations for You. Vulture. May 5, 2019. https://www.vulture. com/2019/05/snl-adam-sandler-is-a-brutally-honest-italian-tour-guide.html

65. Harvard Health. Giving Thanks Can Make You Happier. Blog. Harvard Health Publishing. August 14, 2021. https://www.health.harvard.edu/ healthbeat/giving-thanks-can-make-you-happier#:~:text=In%20positive%20 psychology%20research%2C%20gratitude,adversity%2C%20and%20 build%20strong%20relationships.

66. Robbins T. Neuro-Linguistic Programming Techniques. Blog. Tony Robbins. https://www.tonyrobbins.com/leadership-impact/nlp-techniques/

67. Hornberger T, Wood GS. Benjamin Franklin. Britannica. December 26, 2023. https://www.britannica.com/biography/Benjamin-Franklin/ Achievements-and-inventions

68. Miller GE. 70% of American Want to be Self-Employed. 6% Are. Blog. 20 Something Finance. April 8, 2023. https://20somethingfinance.com/ self-employment-poll/

69. Lennon J. Imagine. Apple Records. AZlyrics.com.. https://www.azlyrics.com/ lyrics/johnlennon/imagine.html

70. Dotson B. Potato Peelers Put Him on Park Avenue. TODAYshow.com. October 2, 2008. https://web.archive.org/web/20100405225806/http://today. msnbc.msn.com/id/26976442/ns/today-today_people

71. Martin E. How One 31-Year-Old Paid Off $220,000 in Student Loans in 3 Years. *Business Insider*. March 8, 2017. https://www.businessinsider. com/how-ebony-horton-paid-off-220000-worth-of-student-loans-in-3-years-2017-3

72. Kachroo-Levine M. This Couple Proves You Can Buy Property and Pay Off $200,000 of Student Loan Debt in 3 Years. *Forbes*. March 23, 2017. https://www.forbes.com/sites/mayakachroolevine/2017/03/23/ this-couple-proves-you-can-buy-property-and-pay-off-200000-of-student-loan-debt-in-3-years/?sh=7d0fbce518b8

73. BBC. The World's Greatest Money Maker: Evan Davis Meets Warren Buffett. TV Movie. BBCTwo. October 27, 2009.

74. CBS. "Person to Person": Warren Buffett. CBS News. November 16, 2012. https://www.cbsnews.com/news/person-to-person-warren-buffett/

75. Kizuna. Ikigai: The Japanese Secret to a Joyful Life. *Kizuna*. March 18, 2022. https://www.japan.go.jp/kizuna/2022/03/ikigai_japanese_secret_to_a_ joyful_life.html

76. United Nations. Once Again, US and Europe Way Ahead on Daily Calorie

Intake. United Nations News. December 12, 2022. https://news.un.org/en/story/2022/12/1131637

77. Worthing B. Extreme Obesity Shaves Years Off Life Expectancy: Four Questions with Dr. Cari Kitahara. Blog. NIH Intramural Research Program. January 23, 2020. https://irp.nih.gov/blog/post/2020/01/extreme-obesity-shaves-years-off-life-expectancy

78. Centers for Disease Control and Prevention. Adult Obesity Facts. Data and Statistics. Centers for Disease Control and Prevention. https://www.cdc.gov/obesity/data/adult.html

79. Detrano J. Sugar Addiction: More Serious Than You Think. Rutgers Center of Alcohol and Substance Abuse Studies. https://alcoholstudies.rutgers.edu/sugar-addiction-more-serious-than-you-think/

80. Jacques A, Chaaya N, Beecher K, Ali SA, Belmer A, Bartlett S. The Impact of Sugar Consumption on Stress Driven, Emotional and Addictive Behaviors. *Neurosci Biobehav Rev*. 2019 Aug;103:178-199. doi: 10.1016/j.neubiorev.2019.05.021. Epub 2019 May 21. PMID: 31125634.

81. Li P, Yin F, Zhao Y, Liu Y, Zhang R, Wang J, Lu W, Wang Q, Zhang J. Total Sugar Intake Is Associated With Higher Prevalence of Depressive Symptoms in Obese Adults. *Front Public Health*. 2023 Jan 13;10:1069162. doi: 10.3389/fpubh.2022.1069162. PMID: 36711384; PMCID: PMC9880186.

82. Engber D. Unexpected Clues Emerge About Why Diets Fail. *Scientific American*. January 13, 2020. https://www.scientificamerican.com/article/unexpected-clues-emerge-about-why-diets-fail/#:~:text=Research%20suggests%20that%20roughly%2080,they%20lose%20within%20two%20years.

83. Campbell-Danesh A. Why Do Most Diets Fail in the Long Run? Blog. *Psychology Today*. August 31, 2020. https://www.psychologytoday.com/us/blog/mind-body-food/202008/why-do-most-diets-fail-in-the-long-run

84. Centers for Disease Control and Prevention. Americans Slightly Taller, Much Heavier Than Four Decades Ago. Press Release. National Center for Health Statistics. October 27, 2004. https://www.cdc.gov/nchs/pressroom/04news/americans.htm

85. Rabin RC. What Foods Are Banned in Europe but Not Banned in the U.S.? The New York Times. December 28, 2018. https://www.nytimes.com/2018/12/28/well/eat/food-additives-banned-europe-united-states.html

86. Garvey M. Meditation Rooms Are the Hottest New Work Perk. MarketWatch. October 26, 2018. https://www.marketwatch.com/story/meditation-rooms-are-the-hottest-new-work-perk-2018-10-26

87. King, C, Goffin G. Up on the Roof. DistroKid, Sony/ATV Music Publishing LLC.

88. U.S. Department of Health and Human Services. Physical Activity Guidelines. U.S. Department of Health and Human Services. https://health.gov/our-work/nutrition-physical-activity/physical-activity-guidelines/current-guidelines

89. Gymless. New Survey Reveals 39.4% of Americans "Never" Exercise; Massive Regional Discrepancies. Press Release. PR Newswire. October 11, 2021. https://www.prnewswire.com/news-releases/new-survey-reveals-39-4-of-americans-never-exercise-massive-regional-discrepancies-301396134.html

90. Paluch AE, Bajpai S, Bassett DR, Carnethon MR, et al. Daily Steps and All-Cause Mortality: A Meta-Analysis of 15 International Cohorts. *The Lancet.* 2022;7(3):E219–E228. https://www.thelancet.com/journals/lanpub/article/PIIS2468-2667(21)00302-9/fulltext

91. Maryville University. Adult Students in Higher Education Statistics. Blog. Maryville University. March 27, 2018. https://online.maryville.edu/blog/going-back-to-school-statistics/

92. Lumina Foundation. https://www.luminafoundation.org/

93. Diaz-Infante N, Lazar M, Ram S, Ray A. Demand for Online Education Is Growing. Are Providers Ready? McKinsey & Company. July 20, 2022. https://www.mckinsey.com/industries/education/our-insights/demand-for-online-education-is-growing-are-providers-ready

94. Guinness. Oldest Graduate. Guiness World Records. https://www.guinnessworldrecords.com/world-records/oldest-graduate

95. U.S. Bureau of Labor Statistics. Labor Force Statistics from the Current Population Survey. U.S. Bureau of Labor Statistics. https://www.bls.gov/cps/cpsaat36.htm

96. AmeriCorps. Formal Volunteering and Informal Helping. AmeriCorps. https://www.americorps.gov/about/our-impact/volunteering-civic-life#:~:text=Formal%20Volunteering,-Formal%20volunteering%20involves&text=An%20estimated%2023.2%20percent%20of,economic%20value%20of%20%24122.9%20billion.

97. Dreyfus SN. Volunteerism and US Civil Society. *Stanford Social Innovation Review.* August 29, 2018. https://ssir.org/articles/entry/volunteerism_and_us_civil_society

98. U.S. Bureau of Labor Statistics. Volunteering in the United States — 2015. Press Release. U.S. Bureau of Labor Statistics. February 25, 2016. https://www.bls.gov/news.release/pdf/volun.pdf

Printed in the USA
CPSIA information can be obtained
at www.ICGtesting.com
CBHW071338050424
6444CB00015B/1347

9 781960 762153